Praise for *Lead*

"This is a very well-written, w

—Bret C. Cormier, *Southeast Missouri State University*

"This book is an intimate, honest and real-world introduction to the use of formative evaluation practices for continuous improvement in a school system. The author's first-hand account provides actionable tools as well as demonstration of their application in practice. The book is both theoretical and applied, which makes it a useful handbook for those who are engaged in continuous improvement of complex systems."

—Dasha Shamrova, *Wichita State University*

"This text teaches change processes through an overarching case example, which makes the concepts more accessible and understandable as students see how things are actually applied."

—John B. Stark, *California State University, Bakersfield*

"This book provides an insightful journey from improvement science through complex system change. The case study presented allows readers to reflect on their own journeys in evaluation and change within the complex systems that we often dismiss."

—Wesley Wilson, *Excalibur Education Group*

"This text uses real-life examples to apply theory and emphasize the important role of continuous improvement in public and nonprofit programs."

—Ryan Yeung, *Hunter College*

Leading Change Through Evaluation

Evaluation in Practice Series - EIPS

Christina A. Christie & Marvin C. Alkin, *Series Editors*

Leading Change Through Evaluation

Improvement Science in Action

Kristen L. Rohanna
University of California

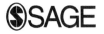

Los Angeles | London | New Delhi
Singapore | Washington DC | Melbourne

FOR INFORMATION:

SAGE Publications, Inc.
2455 Teller Road
Thousand Oaks, California 91320
E-mail: order@sagepub.com

SAGE Publications Ltd.
1 Oliver's Yard
55 City Road
London, EC1Y 1SP
United Kingdom

SAGE Publications India Pvt. Ltd.
B 1/I 1 Mohan Cooperative Industrial Area
Mathura Road, New Delhi 110 044
India

SAGE Publications Asia-Pacific Pte. Ltd.
18 Cross Street #10-10/11/12
China Square Central
Singapore 048423

Library of Congress Cataloging-in-Publication Data

Names: Rohanna, Kristen L., author.

Title: Leading change through evaluation : improvement science in action / Kristen L. Rohanna, University of California.

Description: Los Angeles : SAGE Publications, Inc, [2022] | Includes bibliographical references and index.

Identifiers: LCCN 2021022021 | ISBN 9781071847862 (paperback) | ISBN 9781071847886 (epub) | ISBN 9781071847879 (epub) | ISBN 9781071847893 (ebook)

Subjects: LCSH: Science—Evaluation. | Science—Methodology.

Classification: LCC Q175 .R539 2022 | DDC 001.4/2—dc23

LC record available at https://lccn.loc.gov/2021022021

This book is printed on acid-free paper.

Acquisitions Editor: Helen Salmon
Product Associate: Kenzie Offley
Production Editor: Megha Negi
Copy Editor: Deanna Noga
Typesetter: Hurix Digital
Cover Designer: Scott Van Atta
Marketing Manager: Victoria Velasquez

21 22 23 24 25 10 9 8 7 6 5 4 3 2 1

• Brief Contents •

• Detailed Contents •

• Series Editor Introduction •

Marv Alkin and I set out to produce a book series that takes up new and important trends in evaluation practice. These books are intended not to be general textbooks on the practice of evaluation. Rather, we hope that readers have an opportunity to learn more about a specific topic or approach to evaluation. As scholars who are deeply interested in evaluation theory, we also expect that the books in this series be grounded in theoretical work so that readers have a frame for understanding the rationale for practice decisions. In this book, Rohanna takes a well-recognized framework for improving program and organizational practices in the health fields, known as *improvement science*, and translates it for us into an educational evaluation context. The translation helps broaden improvement science as an evaluative process and widen its application and uses. In this way, it serves as a model for how to traverse multiple intellectual and applied contexts. A first of its kind, there is much to be learned from the empirically grounded work presented in this book, both about the framework that guides her practice as well as from the practice described.

Christina A. Christie

• Acknowledgments •

This book would not be possible without the support of so many people. First, to Christina A. Christie, who first suggested that I turn my dissertation into a book and provided invaluable feedback throughout the research and writing process. Thank you for all the support and guidance. I am deeply grateful to Mike Rose, my writing guru, who guided me through the book writing process. Additionally, I am extremely grateful to my dissertation committee, Christina A. Christie, Louis Gomez, Jim Stigler, Jody Priselac, and Katie Anderson-Levitt, whose thoughtful input helped shape the case study at the heart of this book.

Incredible thanks are owed to the teachers and administrators who participated in the book's networked improvement community. Their dedication, commitment, and desire to improve for their students inspired me every day and encouraged me to do my best, both in my research and the network. Great appreciation is due to Jody Priselac and the hub team, Theodore Sagun, Sarah Bang, June Kim, and Alex Kim. It was a privilege and joy to learn and work with them throughout this project. Special gratitude is also owed to the Carnegie Corporation of New York, whose funding made this important network possible.

I am grateful for feedback from the following reviewers:

- Bret D. Cormier, *Southeast Missouri State University*

- Martha McGuire, *Ryerson University*

- Nahoko Kawakyu O'Connor, *University of Rochester*

- Dasha Shamrova, *Wichita State University*

- John B. Stark, *California State University, Bakersfield*

- Scott D. Tunison, *University of Saskatchewan*

- Gary VanLandingham, *Florida State University*

- Wesley Wilson, *Excalibur Education Group*

- Ryan Yeung, *Hunter College*

- Mariya Yukhymenko, *California State University, Fresno*

Last, to Dara Yueh, who encouraged me to take risks in my writing and spent many hours reviewing my chapters and providing feedback. This book would not be possible without her.

• Foreword •

On matters of seeing, valuing, and understanding the dynamics of change, evaluators get a birds-eye view. The view from the evaluator's perch is presumed to be expansive and holistic. Evaluators see the system of change, the whole, not just its elements. Those not in the evaluator's seat are more likely to see only part of the story. It is difficult to see the inner workings of complex systems. The parable of the six blind men and the elephant that originated on the ancient Indian subcontinent illustrates why it is challenging to see order to the complex problems around us. In the parable, the blind men who have longed to "see" an elephant finally get the opportunity to explore one through touch. The man who touched the elephant's side surmised that the elephant was like a wall. The one who encountered the tusks concluded that an elephant was not all like a wall but a spear. And so, it went with each "seeing" the elephant as something different. This pattern continued as each found a different surface until the sixth blind man found the tail and reckoned that an elephant must be like a rope.

Like the blind men, left to our own devices when faced with complex interventions and programs, we see only part of the value story. Consider what transpires when explaining the success of a new instructional regime. For some people, the impact story is one of the successful materials. For others, it might be the trump of professional development. Others might see it as the power of leadership. Even though evaluation is a relatively young science, policymakers, practitioners, government leaders, and the civic elite have turned to evaluation professionals to help discern holistic substantive value. As interventions and social programs have become more complex, the evaluation and evaluators' importance has become more outsized.

But what counts as the knowledge that offers a holistic appreciation of the inner working of complex systems? The evaluation community's dominant answer has, heretofore, been to identify *what works*. Discerning of substance in this view is encapsulated in knowing how the thing—social program, curriculum, new technology—worked. The evaluation field has behaved as though customers—the aforementioned policymakers, practitioners, government leaders, and civic elites—only have an intellectual appetite for one kind of knowledge: declarative knowledge. The field has behaved as though the customers only want to know the outcome. In short, just the facts, please. The scholarship story ably told in this book by Kristen Rohanna paints a more nuanced picture of the evaluation's customers and clients' intellectual evaluation appetites.

The conceptualization herein Rohanna acknowledges that what works is, of course, important, but she presses the case that the complexity of the whole is better conveyed to clients when they also understand *who* the intervention works for and *in what* contextual settings. In this view, evaluation moves beyond feeding the appetite for declarative knowledge. It also feeds the appetite of the process-centered mind and the relationship-centered mind.

In Rohanna's analysis, seeing the whole also involves shining a bright light on valued procedures uncovered through evaluation inquiry. Procedure-centered understanding goes beyond what we would typically think of as formative investigation. Most formative study aims to find intermediate outcomes, on the way to summary judgment. Rohanna considers processual inquiry and its products a first-class substantive result to be valued in and of itself and not simply a handmaiden to the question of what worked. In a similar vein, the book's inquiry also looks to feed the relationship-centered mind's appetites. Here the examination hews toward understanding how intervention engenders social relationships. Social networks and what strengthens them are also seen as essential outcomes on their own.

In taking this tack, Rohanna joins a growing set of evaluation scholars like Pawson and Tilley (1997) who consider understanding context as a first-class object of evaluation inquiry. She also joins Patton (2016) in taking on the who-is-involved as a vital outcome of evaluation inquiry. This book moves this thinking forward in a fundamental way. Rohanna firmly places continuous improvement generally (Deming, 2018; Langley et al., 2009) and improvement science in particular (Bryk et al., 2015) in the vernacular and conceptual tool kit of evaluation. Why do this? Rohanna gives us at least three reasons. First, continuous improvement offers evaluators a common language to expand into process and relationship. Second, improvement offers the evaluator specific tools to make processes and relationships visible to the evaluation scholarly community and to clients. Third, at its core, quality improvement (Deming, 2018) is about bringing those on the front lines of work (clients and customers) into the web of inquiry. Rohanna takes up the charge pioneered by scholars like Patton (1994) and, more recently, Yurkofsk and colleagues (2020), who conjecture that deep local participation is key to successful evaluation inquiry that has impact. When customers actively join the web of inquiry with the evaluators, together they become more like what Sherer and colleagues (2020) call "analytical partners." One might conjecture that in the analytic partner relationship lies the seeds of resolving an age-old tension. Evaluation scholarship has been fraught by the generalizable rigor—local relevance dilemma. On the one hand, evaluation inquiry demands rigor of the positivist arms-length variety. On the other hand, evaluation inquiry demands local connection and relevance inquiry. The appeal to improvement science provides the field of evaluation with a bridge between methodological rigor and deep respect for context.

I began this foreword, wondering how evaluators might take better advantage of their birds-eye view of change. How might evaluation scholarship help clients have a better vantage point on substantive change? How can evaluation help clients avoid the plight of the blind men in the parable? By and large, most evaluators' answer is telling us what works. Rohanna's book is a fresh salvo in the mix. To wit, she explores techniques that reveal *the who* and *the how* as objects of inquiry. I suspect this work will come to be seen as an essential contribution to evaluation scholarship.

Louis Gomez,
University of California, Los Angeles
April 2021

• Preface •

Evaluation can be a powerful lever for social change. Today's persistent problems often exist in complex systems, whether it be a school district addressing high rates of chronic absenteeism or a hospital investigating why a high number of patients are acquiring new infections in their care. Improving these societal challenges requires continuous, systematic, and systemic inquiry. Evaluation provides methods to guide this inquiry.

As evaluators interested in leading change, we often turn to formative evaluation approaches without really understanding their distinctions or how one is more suitable for our needs than another. Based on my experience, it is not uncommon to hear evaluators ask how and why different formative evaluation models are unique. Rather than being a catch-all term for disciplined inquiry aimed at program and policy development or improvement, formative evaluation approaches need to be more formally systematized based on their intended uses. That is, not all formative evaluation models have the same purpose. This lack of use specificity can lead evaluators to question which approach will work best for their specific needs. In practice, an evaluator might wonder, "Should I use Developmental Evaluation, or Improvement Science, or a more general use-oriented formative approach?" I know, because I have been that evaluator.

Leading Change Through Evaluation takes a deeper dive. It expands on why those hoping to use evaluation to drive change in complex systems—rather than develop or improve one program, policy, or product—need to shift from the oversimplified idea of formative evaluation to a more specified continuous improvement model grounded in improvement science. In doing so, this book provides guidance to both evaluators and others, such as K–12 educators and hospital administrators, who lead improvement initiatives in their organizations and seek to solve persistent problems of practice.

This book is organized into two parts. Part 1 (Chapters 1–2) provides the necessary background for understanding the concepts of persistent problems, formative evaluation, continuous improvement and improvement science, and complexity science and systems thinking. Part 2 (Chapters 3–8) offers an empirical case study as an example of evaluation in practice. Other books provide principles, tenets, or methods for improvement; this book is unique because it provides a real-world example of leading a network improvement initiative in five secondary schools committed to improving student learning in math. As such, it unpacks how to build teachers' capacity to engage in improvement, including details about the practical challenges. Importantly, this book provides an in-depth look at how and why particular decisions were made by those leading the endeavor. The last chapter summarizes the lessons learned through this case study, including a new conceptualized improvement capacity-building model for others leading similar change initiatives.

It is important to be forthcoming about my positionality. This book was born out of my dissertation, which I wrote in the summer of 2018. I was part of the team from a Southern California university who coordinated the improvement network at the heart of this book's case study. As part of that team, I was responsible for planning, facilitating, and leading improvement science activities in the network. My positionality posed benefits and challenges while conducting this study. While it provided me access to all network-related meetings and decisions, enabling me to write a detailed narrative, my positionality also impacted my research. That is, my research lens was that of an insider rather than an outsider. This insider perspective, combined with primarily qualitative data, subjected my research to potential biases. As such, I took steps to address this issue. I attended to my reflexivity throughout the study. I collected and triangulated data from multiple sources, systematically considered alternative hypotheses and disconfirming evidence, and engaged in peer debriefing and member checks with others. I further validated my findings by comparing them to similar research (Proger, Bhatt, Cirks, & Gurke, 2017).

Notably, this positioning gave me a unique insight into leading evaluative and improvement initiatives for change. This book shares my experiences and learnings. It is written for other evaluators and practitioners hoping to lead change and solve society's most persistent challenges. Those seeking to learn more about evaluation and leadership may find this book helpful both as example in practice and empirical research on evaluation and improvement processes. While this book includes many examples from education, it also incorporates content from other disciplines and the lessons can be applied broadly. The book draws on evaluation, organizational learning, complexity science, and adult and workplace learning theories. Readers are encouraged to make connections to their own practice and contexts through end-of-chapter discussion questions. I hope this book will guide others as they seek to effect positive change in the world.

• About the Author •

Kristen Rohanna is a professor in the Educational Leadership Program and Social Research Methodology Division in the School of Education and Information Studies at the University of California, Los Angeles (UCLA). Rohanna's practice and research focus on using evaluative methods to effect social change, with a particular emphasis in the area of education. As such, she works closely with K–12 teachers and administrators to support their use of evaluation and improvement science methods. Before her time at UCLA, Rohanna was a Harvard Strategic Data Fellow and the Manager for Research and Evaluation at the San Jose Unified School District. The experience provided the context for her *New Direction for Evaluation* article: "Breaking the Adopt, Attack, Abandon Cycle: A Case for Improvement Science in K–12 Education," about the potential power of continuous improvement methods and the challenges school leaders face when attempting to undertake these methods. Rohanna also has a forthcoming article in the *American Journal of Evaluation* about building the improvement science capacity of teachers.

Rohanna has extensive program evaluation experience, including leading numerous program evaluations for the California Department of Education. Currently, she is leading a statewide evaluation of the 21st Century California School Leadership Academy. The initiative provides professional learning opportunities to K–12 education leaders, including equity-centered leadership and improvement science.

Rohanna received her Bachelor of Arts degree in History from the University of Pittsburgh and her Master of Arts degree in Demographic and Social Analysis from the University of California, Irvine. She received her PhD in Social Research Methodology from UCLA.

Seeking Change in a Complex World

In the mid-1970s, Ernö Rubik created a puzzle that he could not easily solve. He was a professor at the Academy of Applied Arts in Budapest Hungary and wanted a tool to help his students learn three-dimensional geometry and movement (Simpson, 2015; Wallop, 2014). Using materials found in his mother's home, he designed a cube-shaped model with nine primary color squares on each side. He named it the "Magic Cube." Now, he was stumped. As he moved one side, another side would move. The movement of one colored square influenced the movement of another square. With each move, the brightly colored squares became more jumbled. There were 43 quintillion possible permutations. It took him a month to solve it.

If you are a child of the 1980s, you probably remember trying your hand at Rubik's Cube. If you were like me, you couldn't do it. A few of our fellow Generation Xers got creative and tried a different approach: They simply pried off the jumbled color pieces and re-glued them to match on each side. Problem solved! Or was it?

What those industrious Generation Xers might not remember, or perhaps never knew, was that by taking the cube apart and rebuilding it, you could actually render the puzzle unsolvable. Rubik's Cube purists will tell you that scrambling the pieces throws off the orientations of the edge and corners pieces. It is a system of interconnected pieces.

Three decades later, communities across the United States were facing a puzzle of a different, more dangerous sort. In 2018, there were approximately 47,000 opioid overdose deaths in the United

States (Centers for Disease Control and Prevention [CDC], 2020a). Opioid use was not a new epidemic. Between 1999 and 2018, the number of opioid-related deaths had increased drastically (CDC, 2020a). Numerous federal, state, and local efforts had been undertaken for years to improve the problem. Promising solutions were known. For instance, the state of Washington passed prescription reform legislation that resulted in a "27 percent reduction in the number of overdose deaths between 2008 and 2012" (Martin et al., 2016, p. 6).

However, as legislative efforts addressed the over-prescription of opioids, new problems emerged, creating three waves of opioid overdose deaths (CDC, 2020b). The first wave of deaths occurred because of the rise of prescription opioids in the 1990s. The second wave began around 2010 due to increased heroin use. And the third wave, beginning in 2013 with the sharpest increase, was the result of synthetic opioids such as fentanyl. As prescription abuse decreased, illicit use increased. As law enforcement battled heroin trafficking, fentanyl was introduced. Like a Rubik's Cube with life and death consequences, a change in one area led to a consequence in another. The problem was always changing and thus, remained persistent, and the solution remained elusive.

How does one approach problems in today's complex society? Solving persistent and difficult problems requires a systematic and systemic approach that helps us make continuous moves toward improving the problem. One intervention, one new program, one policy change is unlikely to solve the problem on its own.

During the first wave of opioid crisis, there were numerous interventions that were shown to be effective; however, many were not systemic or continuous. That is, they did not account for the next problem that would arise, whether due to an unintended consequence or another change in the system's landscape. According to an Institute for Healthcare Improvement, the lack of a systems-wide view of the problem was one of the most significant drivers of the crisis (Martin et al., 2016). Among others, they identified these reasons for why the crisis continued:

- Lack of coordination of approaches and resources: They noted that many of the intervention initiatives were siloed and only addressed one part of the problem.

- Lack of effective implementation of promising practices: They suggested that the continued crisis was not due to the lack of knowledge, evidence-based strategies, and recommendations for action, but rather the lack of support for executing these strategies and recommendations.

- Failure to engage necessary communities and stakeholders: Importantly, they acknowledged that improvement efforts needed to include those they intended to help—members of the local communities, families, individuals—along with law enforcement, faith-based organizations, and schools.

As evaluators seeking to lead change, we can easily fall victim to the above failures by focusing on individual interventions, programs, and policies rather than the problem as it exists in a multifaceted complex system.

Part 1 of this book provides a foundational grounding by introducing formative evaluation, continuous improvement, and systems and complexity science theory. Evaluators commonly look to formative evaluation as a guiding framework for change or improvement. Yet to lead change in complex systems, evaluators need to distinguish formative approaches that embrace and provide methods for understanding and being responsive to emerging challenges and complexity.

What do we really mean by formative evaluation? It holds a different meaning for different people. Some consider formative evaluation the first step toward a more conclusive summative evaluation. Others use the term as a catch-all phrase for any evaluation aimed at improvement. Chapter 1 of this book provides the history of formative evaluation and unpacks its different meanings in an effort to help evaluators better specify which model best fits their needs. I further posit that evaluators hoping to improve persistent problems in complex systems should consider continuous improvement approaches grounded in improvement science.

Many of us in evaluation are familiar with the idea of continuous improvement. It takes various forms but is generally considered to be any ongoing endeavor to improve products, processes, practices, or services. While continuous improvement is often regarded as a form of formative evaluation, primarily labeling it so can lead to a potential oversight of its defining characteristic; that continuous improvement is, well, *continuous*. There is no end point to the process. More than a broad formative approach for improving one particular program, policy, or practice, continuous improvement lends itself to an evaluative strategy for driving change in complex systems because it is responsive to emergent challenges.

In Chapter 2, I further consider the concept of complex systems by providing background on complexity theory and systems thinking. Like the social systems in which the opioid crisis exists, today's organizations continually confront challenges, whether it be a school district addressing high rates of chronic absenteeism, or a hospital investigating why a high number of patients are acquiring new infections in their care. These organizations exist in complex systems with many interrelated and dependent parts. The actions of one individual, department, or policy influence other people and processes elsewhere in the system. Furthermore, these actions and related outcomes may be unforeseen because system actors adapt to changes and new contextual conditions resulting from this interconnectedness.

Conditions are rarely stable or predictable. Those hoping to solve persistent problems need to engage and honor the experiences and perspectives of those within the system and build their capacity for ongoing disciplined inquiry. By doing so, those on the front lines are empowered to continually identify and respond to emerging issues. Leading change in complex systems requires a philosophical shift in how people work and learn. This book provides practical guidance in how to build this capacity.

Through an in-depth case study in Part 2, I examine the use of continuous improvement as an evaluative strategy in practice and describe how one approach grounded in improvement science was integrated into an improvement network consisting of five schools who hoped to improve mathematics instruction. By doing so, I provide an empirical example of implementing some of the concepts introduced in Part 1, and importantly, share struggles and difficulties that emerged through the process.

Improvement science is a disciplined inquiry process by which the subject matter and the improvement experts (often the evaluator) collaborate to find the root cause of a problem within a system, develop a theory of change for improving it, and rapidly experiment with changes to determine if they lead to improvements. This book's case study addresses real-world improvement science challenges and complexities rather than solely sharing the ideal situation. Instead of directing how the process should be in the ideal context, I discuss what it looks like in an actual context then encapsulate the case study's significant learnings and offer additional lessons learned since researching the case study.

My hope is that this book provides practical guidance to other evaluators seeking to effect positive change in the world. It is a call to action.

Change is hard. Change is messy. Change is hardest and messiest in complex systems where one can't simply force the pieces to fit the solution like a re-glued Rubik's Cube. But change is not impossible if evaluators and practitioners add the right tools to their toolbox. This book offers some of those tools.

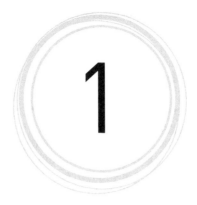

What Do We Mean by Formative Evaluation?

I became interested in improvement science early in my graduate school career. As a program evaluator in a PhD program, others often asked me how improvement science differed from formative evaluation and developmental evaluation. At the time I did not have good answer. Now, I do.

Purpose distinguishes the approach. This foundational chapter begins our journey of understanding how to lead change through evaluation by delving into the meaning of formative evaluation and how it has evolved over the years. It sets the stage for why continuous improvement methods (e.g., improvement science as a form of formative evaluation) are a valuable approach for driving change in complex systems.

In this chapter, I cover:

- The Evolution of Formative Evaluation

- Continuous Improvement and Improvement Science

- Other Continuous Improvement Approaches

The Evolution of Formative Evaluation

Evaluators often find themselves in one of two broad roles: providing a credible and balanced summative judgment about a program or policy, or formatively supporting the development or improvement of some program, policy, process, or organizational practice. Evaluators conducting summative evaluations engage in systematic inquiry to provide a conclusion about an entity's worth or effectiveness and typically provide findings to stakeholders at the end of an evaluation. Those involved in formative evaluation also engage in systematic inquiry, but the process is designed to deliver timelier data and findings to inform stakeholders about what or how to improve. Both roles are important and can be used for improvement, but this chapter focuses on the latter, using formative evaluation as an evaluative strategy to lead change.

Michael Scriven introduced the term "formative evaluation" in the late 1960s. In *The Methodology of Evaluation* (1966), he importantly distinguished the *goals* of evaluation from the *roles* of evaluation. His paper focused on curricular evaluation, although his points also applied to other kinds of evaluation. Scriven stated that the *goals* of evaluation were to answer questions about how well "certain entities" perform, either on their own, or compared to another (p. 2). The *roles* of evaluation, however, could take various forms. To use Scriven's examples, evaluation could play a role in the development of curriculum or in determining the worth of that curriculum. By making this argument, he distinguished "formative" evaluation aimed at improving a program during its development, from "summative" evaluation that sought to provide final conclusions about a program's value or worth.

Notably, Scriven was arguing a counterpoint to Cronbach (1963), who viewed course improvement as a *primary* purpose of evaluation. Cronbach also focused on education and curriculum, and in this context, improvement meant "deciding what instructional materials and methods are satisfactory and where change is needed" (p. 236).[1] Cronbach posited that "the greatest service evaluation can perform is to identify aspects of the course where revision is desirable" (p. 238) and that "evidence must become available midway in curriculum development . . ." (p. 239). He stated that "[e]valuation, used to improve the course while it is still fluid, contributes more to improvement of education than evaluation used to appraise a product already placed on the market" (p. 239). While Scriven (1966, 1996) believed that formative evaluations were valuable and necessary, they were not a substitute for a final summary judgment about a course or program. Both were important roles of evaluation. For Scriven, and subsequently many other evaluators, improvement was formative evaluation, and its primary purpose was as a step toward preparing a program for a subsequent summative evaluation, not for the sake of improvement itself. Thus, he coined the terms formative and summative evaluation to make a distinction between the two.

However, the meaning of formative evaluation has evolved over the years. Many evaluators use the term to mean any type of evaluative activity aimed at improving a policy, program, or process, and not solely as a step toward preparing them for a summative evaluation. Yet for some evaluators, it is Scriven's initial viewpoint of formative evaluation that prevents them from embracing

---

[1]Cronbach also listed two other types of decisions for which evaluation is used: (1) "Decisions about individuals: identifying the needs of the pupil for the sake of planning his instruction, judging pupil merit for purposes of selection and grouping, acquainting the pupil with his own progress and deficiencies." (2) "Administrative regulation: judging how good the school system is, how good individual teachers are, etc." (p. 236).

the term more broadly. For example, in 1996, Michael Quinn Patton, a well-known evaluator and former president of the American Evaluation Association, acknowledged that the meaning of formative evaluation "has been enlarged to include any evaluation whose primary purpose is program improvement" (p. 135). However, in that same article, he stopped short of claiming that developmental evaluation was a form of formative evaluation because its purpose was not to prepare for a summative evaluation. Developmental evaluation is an evaluation model that seeks to *develop* innovative programs, products, policy reforms, and organizational changes in complex environments (Patton, 2011). Scriven's definition at the time was too limiting.

Even since then, the concept of formative evaluation has continued to progress and become a catch-all term synonymous with evaluation for improvement. This is, at the very least, partially due to the expanding discipline of evaluation in which there are multiple models and approaches of evaluation that extend beyond Scriven's original dichotomy of formative and summative. However, the concept of what formative evaluation means is still vague.

For some, formative evaluation's purpose is to improve the program, typically as part of understanding implementation or processes before evaluating whether the program is achieving intended outcomes.

In *Evaluation Essentials*, Alkin and Vo (2018) provide this definition of formative evaluation:

> *Formative evaluation* generally takes place during the early stages of program implementation. Formative evaluation is conducted in order to provide information for program improvement, which generally means that the evaluation information would provide an indication of how things are going. (p. 12, emphasis in original)

While Alkin and Vo (2018) seem to subscribe to the more traditional definition of formative evaluation, they also acknowledge that formative evaluation may "take place over extended periods of time" and label this as *continuous* formative evaluation, which is "focused on the ongoing development of a program or innovation in more complex settings" (p. 12). They note that some call this practice "developmental evaluation," thereby either acknowledging a broader conception of formative evaluation or a potential divergence from Patton (1996) on whether developmental evaluation falls under the formative umbrella.

Further, Alkin and Vo (2018) provide another important distinction within the category of formative evaluation: Evaluators only occasionally conduct *final* summative evaluations. Rather, evaluators more often practice what they call "summary formative evaluation" (p. 13). There may be a period of time where formative activities occur, and then the evaluator will summarize findings at the end of that period. Additionally, Alkin and Vo remind us that both processes and interim outcomes (versus end-of-evaluation outcomes) may be included in summary formative evaluations. Many use summary results for program improvement, and many summarize formative results to reach conclusions. And, in fact, it is the use of the information that determines its categorization.

There is a classic maxim in evaluation attributed to Robert Stake:

- When the cook tastes the soup, that's formative.
- When the guest tastes the soup, that's summative.

Alkin and Vo (2018) further this idea by considering that (1) when the cook tastes the soup, they are interested in whether it tastes good (interim summary outcome), and (2) when the guest tastes the soup, the cook may also be interested in the guest's feedback for the purpose of improving the soup the next time they serve it (summary formative evaluation).

Expanding on their ideas, now consider: Should the cook ever stop caring whether the guest likes the soup? Even if the recipe does not change, the context might. Restaurant menus of the 1970s commonly offered pea soup, but today, the humble pea soup has been replaced by carrot ginger, cucumber gazpacho, miso, and other recipes preferred by today's palates. Also, consider the scenario where the restaurant's management changes. The old cook is replaced by a new chef. Might this change how the soup recipe is implemented and subsequently tastes in this new context? Summary conclusions can be ongoing and responsive to the latest needs.

What is considered formative or summative depends on the purpose, use, and context. Scriven (1996) himself made this point. Therefore, extending the concept of formative evaluation more broadly makes practical sense. As Alkin and Vo mention, only occasionally do program designers, staff, and evaluators stop at a final assessment of the program's value or worth.

Many of today's evaluation needs are formative and *ongoing*. That is, programs aimed at improving particular societal problems can rarely afford to remain static. What once worked, or worked in a particular context, may not work again. Let us return to the persistent problem of opioid overdoses discussed earlier. As progress was made in the first wave of deaths due to prescription painkillers, another challenge soon emerged in the form of heroin abuse. When progress was made combatting heroin use, a new problem arose: fentanyl. The Institute for Healthcare Improvement (Martin et al., 2016) suggested that this problem does not persist due to a lack of knowledge, evidence-based strategies, and recommendations. Rather, one of the reasons is a lack of effective implementation of these strategies and recommendations. Consistent implementation is often a challenge in any context, yet in a complex environment where people, policies, and places are never static, the challenge of implementation is multifaceted.

If we return to Alkin and Vo's (2018) definition of formative evaluation—"formative evaluation generally takes place during the early stages of program implementation"—responding to the emergent challenges arising while implementing a potential solution is formative. And if an evaluator is *continually* addressing emergent needs in the pursuit of improving a program, policy, or problem, they are engaged in formative evaluation regardless of whether the intervention ever reaches the summative state because in complex environments with persistent problems, one can rarely reach the stable environment conducive to a conclusive summative evaluation. Instead, evaluators are often engaged in continuous formative evaluation to respond to program development in complex settings (Alkin and Vo, 2018). Complex persistent problems require agility and responsiveness to emergent evidence by program designers *and* evaluators.

Patton (2011) provided an example of this necessity in the opening pages of his book *Developmental Evaluation: Applying Complexity Concepts to Enhance Innovation and Use*. He described the moment when developmental evaluation, as a specific model of evaluation, was born. As an evaluation consultant working with a community leadership program in Minnesota, his 5-year contract specified a need for 2 1/2 years of formative evaluation services, followed by 2 1/2 years of summative evaluation services. The first phase went well. Patton explained how the program made major programmatic and operational changes as part of the formative evaluation, and program staff enthusiastically sought feedback to continually make improvements. Then came the moment to transition from the formative evaluation to the summative.

As Patton detailed in his book, he began to see a shift in the group:

We've had a couple of years changing and adapting the program. I've been impressed by your openness and commitment to use evaluation feedback to make improvements. But now, in the next phase of the evaluation, called summative evaluation, the purpose is to make an overall judgment about the merit and worth of the program. Does it work? Should it be continued, perhaps even expanded? Have you come up with a model that others might want to adopt? This means that from now on you can't make any more improvements or changes because we need the program—the model—to stay stable in order to conduct the summative evaluation. Only with a fixed intervention, carefully implemented the same way for each new group of leaders in training, can we attribute the measured outcomes to your program intervention in a valid and credible way.

Mouths fell open. Staff was aghast. They protested:

We don't want to implement a fixed model. In fact, what we've learned is that we need to keep adapting what we do to the particular needs of new groups. Communities vary. The backgrounds of our participants vary. The economic and political context keeps changing. New technologies like the Internet are coming into rural Minnesota and creating new leadership challenges. Small communities are becoming parts of regional networks. We need to get more young people into the program. Immigrants are moving into rural Minnesota in droves, creating more diverse communities. We need to reach out and adapt what we do to Native Americans. No! No! No! We can't fix the model. We can't stand still for 2 years. We don't want to do the summative evaluation. (p. 2)

Patton described the rest of the conversation with the group and the eventual agreement that they would never conduct a summative evaluation on this program. Rather, it would remain in a constant *developmental* stage and they would continually report their activities, developments, and learnings to stakeholders. And there, according to Patton, he coined the term "developmental evaluation."

In addition to the program staff recognizing the need for a new evaluation approach to respond to their community's complexity, it is notable that Patton was still bounded by traditional notions of evaluation. That is, to justify a continuous formative approach to evaluation, the program must be considered to be in a perpetual state of development.

Today, formative evaluation has progressed into the broader catch-all term for program improvement. This book subscribes to that broader definition, and thus, considers developmental evaluation as a form of formative evaluation. Yet not all formative evaluation is the same. Different approaches can be further specified by their intended improvement purpose and use. For example, in the case of developmental evaluation, its intended purpose is program development.

Furthermore, broader ideas have evolved around what we consider to be evaluation. Preskill and Torres (1999) extended our notion of what can be evaluated when they advanced Evaluative Inquiry for learning in organizations. They envisioned "evaluative inquiry as an ongoing process for investigating and understanding critical organizational issues" and "an approach to learning that is fully integrated with an organization's work practices" (p. 1). Russ-Eft and Preskill (2009) further cemented these ideas with their characterization of evaluation:

First, evaluation is viewed as a systematic process. It should not be conducted as an afterthought; rather it is a planned and purposeful activity. Second, evaluation involves collecting data regarding questions or issues about society in general and organizations and programs in particular. Third, evaluation is seen as a process for enhancing knowledge and decision making, whether the decisions are related to improving or refining a program, process, product, system, or organization, or determining whether to continue or expand a program. In each of these decisions, there is some aspect of judgment about the evaluand's merit, worth, or value. Finally, the notion of evaluation use is either implicit or explicit in each of the above definitions. (p. 4)

Their third point is especially germane here: Evaluation is seen as a process for enhancing knowledge and decision making, *whether the decisions are related to improving or refining a program, process, product, system, or organization.* Thus, they promote the idea that it is the entity upon which decisions are made that defines the evaluand (i.e., the entity being evaluated). This is broader than more common notions of program, process, product (or policy) and includes a system or organization. Evaluators are no longer limited to Scriven's early proclamation that the goals of evaluation were to answer questions about how well "certain entities" perform. Now, we can embrace the idea that evaluation includes enhancing knowledge and decisions about improvement.

Recently, Rohanna and Christie (in preparation) further expanded the concept of the evaluand by advancing the idea that the evaluation entity can be the social problem within a complex system. By doing so, they build on Preskill and Torres' (1999) and Russ-Eft and Preskill's (2009) ideas that evaluation is a process for investigating organizational issues and enhancing knowledge and decision making to improve a system.

Continuous Improvement and Improvement Science

By subscribing to Russ-Eft and Preskill's description of evaluation, we can embrace continuous improvement as a form of evaluation, and in particular, a type of formative evaluation. However, it is important not to fuse all improvement-oriented approaches under the broad umbrella of formative evaluation. Formative evaluation approaches should be distinguished from each other by their specified use and purpose. Like developmental evaluation, which declares program development as its intended use, continuous improvement has an intended use to *continually* evaluate and improve some entity, whether program, process, product, system, organization, or problem. Its defining characteristic—it is continuous—makes it a promising evaluation strategy for leading change in complex systems, particularly when we consider persistent problems such as the opioid crisis. Notably, continuous improvement approaches can be further specified by their purpose, as discussed later in this chapter.

But first, let us consider another persistent social problem in a complex system: completion rates in California community colleges.

Persistent Social Problems

In her 2013 article titled *Improving on the American Dream,* Gay Clyburn shared the story of Mary Lowry, a student at Foothill College who remembered crying and blaming herself because she could not pass her college math class. An otherwise successful student in high school, Mary had difficulty with math and was placed in a non-credit remedial math course in community college. She struggled. "I thought something was wrong with me," she said. "No matter how hard I tried—and I had really tried hard—I could not pass a math class"

(Clyburn, 2013, p. 15). Mary feared she would not be able to earn her degree, after failing her math class three times.

Like many community college students, Mary was at risk for dropping out of college and not realizing her dreams. In 2013, fewer than half (48.5%) of California community college students completed a degree, certificate, or transferred to a 4-year college within 6 years.[2] Students like Mary who entered community college but deemed unprepared were placed in non-credit remedial courses, also called *developmental courses*. For those students, the completion rate was even lower at 41.1%.

This was a societal problem without an easy fix. California had, and still has, the largest community college system in the United States, serving approximately 2.1 million students across 116 colleges (California Community Colleges Chancellor's Office, 2020a). Most of the students (80%) were enrolled in at least one developmental course during their college experience (Mejia, Rodriguez, & Johnson, 2016). Furthermore, Latinx and African American students were disproportionately affected with higher enrollment in developmental courses, and lower than overall completion rates (CCC Student Success Scorecard; Mejia et al., 2016).

Community colleges are promoted as an affordable, accessible, and equitable path for students to achieve a higher education degree or vocational certificate. More than half of all undergraduate Latinx and African American students attend community college, and many are low-income and nontraditional students (Mejia et al., 2016). Developmental courses were designed to help students who were identified as underprepared for their pursuit of higher learning or a vocational career. The developmental sequence was supposed to provide foundational and basic skills in math or English, and thus help them complete their college-level courses.

The espoused vision of the community college system was "making sure students from all backgrounds succeed in reaching their goals" (California Community Colleges Chancellor's Office, 2020b). In actuality, the system was creating a roadblock by requiring a lengthy developmental sequence and adding multiple semesters of additional coursework for no college credit. The result: Fewer than half of these students actually completed community college. The system was having the opposite effect, and students like Mary were paying the price.

Why? Because requiring developmental courses was an attempt at a straightforward solution to a complex systemic problem. Students who were often identified as underprepared tended to be low-income or nontraditional. They were required to take more classes. More classes meant more tuition costs and greater financial burden. More classes also meant more chances of failure. More failure meant students like Mary blamed themselves rather than the system. Students were failing, giving up, and dropping out.

---

[2] Source: California Community Colleges Student Success Scorecard. Percentage of 2007–2008 cohort who were enrolled the first time and tracked for six years. 5-yr. Trends. https://scorecard.cccco.edu/scorecardrates.aspx?CollegeID=000#home

The problem was difficult to improve. For years, community colleges had been concerned about their low completion rates. State policymakers flowed funding into a multitude of initiatives, including $20 million annually since the 2007–2008 school year for its Basic Skills Initiative (Mejia et al., 2016). Still, the problem persisted.

The Carnegie Foundation for the Advancement of Teaching took a new approach. In 2010, they convened a network of researchers, practitioners, and community college faculty to jointly unpack, frame, and really understand the problem before they set out to solve it (Clyburn, 2013). They developed a new pathway for students placed into developmental math. Students could take a quantitative reasoning (Quantway) or statistics (Statway) course that was both developmental and college-level, allowing them to earn college credit. Additionally, the courses connected math concepts to real-world problems.

But the network did not stop there. Their team of scholarly and practical experts committed to continually studying, understanding, and improving this problem. They developed and tested activities designed to help students persist through the courses and increase their sense of belonging. In their first year, 51% of the 1,077 students enrolled in the Statway course completed the sequence in one semester, compared with 21% of their campus peers who took the traditional path to completing the sequence, which took a year (Silva & White, 2013). Mary was one of those successful Statway students (Clyburn, 2013).

With their success, the Carnegie Foundation continued to roll out the pathway options to more community colleges. Their network committed to continuing their inquiry as they scaled up the pathways. They learned from both what was working well and what could still be improved. By 2016–2017, approximately 7,500 students over 48 institutions were enrolled in either Statway or Quantway, with most of them successfully completing (62% and 72%, respectively) (Huang, 2018).

Although these innovative pathways were working, not all community college students had the opportunity to enroll. In 2017, California policymakers passed Assembly Bill 705, which required colleges to give students alternate options to remedial courses, allow them to enroll in transfer-level courses, and use high school records instead of less predictive placement tests. Early evidence suggests more students are enrolling in non-remedial courses and are succeeding (Mejia, Rodriguez, & Johnson, 2019). Thus, these changes have the potential to disrupt the old system and will require ongoing disciplined inquiry by policymakers, practitioners, researchers, and evaluators to learn from, and respond to, emergent challenges.

The community college example not only serves as an illustration of a persistent problem in a complex system, but it also shows the power of embracing continuous improvement approaches and multiple perspectives for understanding and improving a problem. The Carnegie Foundation for the Advancement of Teaching grounded their network in improvement science.

Improvement Science

The American Society for Quality (ASQ) defines continuous improvement as "the ongoing improvement of products, services or processes through incremental and breakthrough improvements."[3] There are many different models of continuous improvement, including improvement science (i.e., the "science of improvement") (Berwick, 2008, p. 1182). But what exactly does the science of improvement mean? Improvement science is a broad approach with various definitions and models. When it is applied *continuously* as part of an effort to integrate its tools and methods into an organization's everyday work, it falls under the umbrella of continuous improvement; yet, importantly, the two terms are not interchangeable.

Improvement science has been defined as the following:

A field of study focused on the methods, theories, and approaches that facilitate or hinder efforts to improve quality in context-specific work processes, and centers inquiry on the day-to-day 'problems of practice that have genuine consequences for people's lives.' (Bryk, 2009, cited by Park, Hironaka, Carver, & Nordstrum, 2013, p. 598; Health Foundation, 2011).

A data-driven change process that aims to systematically design, test, implement, and scale change toward systemic improvement, as informed and defined by the experience and knowledge of subject matter experts (Lemire, Christie, & Inkelas, 2017, p. 25).

Improvement science is a methodological framework that is undergirded by foundational principals that guide scholar-practitioners to define problems, understand how the system produces the problems, identify changes to rectify the problems, test the efficacy of those changes, and spread the changes (if the change is indeed an improvement) (Hinnant-Crawford, 2020, p. 29).

Improvement science is scientific: It is disciplined and systematic and grounded in a theoretical and methodological approach. It is systemic: It not only seeks to improve a problem but also the system in which the problem is situated. There is substantial overlap between continuous improvement and improvement science. In fact there is so much overlap that differences between the two may seem inconsequential. However, it is important to understand the distinguishing features of each when leading change in complex systems. Not all continuous improvement approaches are scientific or systemic, and not all improvement science is continuous. In my own experiences, I have heard organizations claim they are committed to continuous improvement and implement regular surveys to receive and respond to feedback. There is nothing wrong with this. It is a beneficial, systematic practice for continually improving and meeting stakeholder needs, but it does not address a specific problem situated within a broader system, nor it is grounded in theoretical principles for

---

[3] https://asq.org/quality-resources/quality-glossary/c

improvement. On the flipside, improvement science, while iterative and continuous in its approach to improving a specific problem, does not necessarily instill a continuous improvement culture throughout an organization. There may be one *project* team focused on solving one problem. Once the problem is vastly improved, the team may disband, and along with it, the continuous and collaborative mode for ongoing inquiry. Again, there is nothing wrong with this approach. But the sweet spot is found in the overlap, where inquiry is disciplined and ongoing, embraces a systemic view, and is grounded in theoretical and methodological principles of improvement. Therefore, this book advocates a continuous improvement model that is grounded in improvement science.

Improvement science was founded on much of the work of W. Edward Deming (Langley et al., 2009). Deming was an engineer and statistician who advanced production, management effectiveness, and quality improvement. His ideas shaped Japanese manufacturing and industrial practices after World War II (Walton, 1986).

Improvement science delineates two types of knowledge: subject knowledge and profound knowledge. Subject knowledge is considered the content knowledge within a particular area, often held by practitioners and/or researchers, while profound knowledge is the more systematic awareness of "how to make changes that will result in improvement in a variety of settings" (Langley et al., 2009, p. 75). Deming defined profound knowledge "as the interplay of theories of systems, variation, knowledge, and psychology" (Deming, as cited in Langley et al., 2009, p. 75).

BOX 1.1

Deming structured his system of profound knowledge around four types of knowledge (Christie, Inkelas, & Lemire, 2017):

1. **Knowledge of systems**: This type of knowledge refers to the interdependence of departments, people, and processes within an organization (Langley et al., 2009). Integration of these individual parts toward a common aim contributes to a successful organization (Deming, 1994; Langley et al., 2009).

2. **Knowledge of variation**: This component not only promotes the shift from analyzing averages to a deeper study of variation in data, but it also encourages an understanding of different types of variation and their implications for system performance (Christie, Inkelas, & Lemire, 2017; Langley et al., 2009).

3. **Knowledge of how knowledge grows**: This type of knowledge refers to learning by making predictions about potential changes, then actually making the changes and measuring the results (Langley et al., 2009).

4. **Knowledge of psychology**: This component reflects the human side of change and encompasses how attention to people's values, attitudes, and motivations can influence change (Langley et al., 2009).

Deming is also credited with the Plan, Do, Study, Act (PDSA) cycle, which was an evolution of Walter A. Shewhart's initial cycle of scientific testing (Moen & Norman, 2010). The PDSA cycle is formatted for rapidly experimenting with new practices and generating new knowledge (Langley et al., 2009). Its four stages—plan, do, study, and act—follow a dynamic, deductive, and inductive learning process. Experiment logistics are planned during the first stage (Plan), implemented during the second stage (Do). During the third stage (Study), the experimenter analyzes relevant data, reflects on the process, and determines the next steps. In the final stage (Act) next steps are put into action. Ideally, the PDSA cycle should occur within a short timeframe, on a small scale so ideas can be quickly tested, and either adapted and retested, gradually scaled up, or potentially abandoned as necessary.

From Plan to Do, the deductive approach is applied. A theory is tested with the aid of a prediction. In the Do phase, observations are made and departures from the prediction are noted. From Do to Study, the inductive learning process takes over. Gaps in the prediction are studied and the theory is updated accordingly. Action is then taken on the new learning in the last stage (Langley et al., 2009, p. 82)

Langley and his colleagues (2009) at Associates in Process Improvement expanded on Deming's work and developed the "Model for Improvement." The Model for Improvement encompasses three questions and the PDSA Cycle (Langley et al., 2009). The three questions are:

1. What are we trying to accomplish?

2. How will we know the change is an improvement?

3. What change can we make that will result in an improvement?

While there are different models of improvement science, the process typically encompasses three broad phases illustrated by Figure 1.2. These three stages loosely correspond with the Model for Improvement's three questions.

FIGURE 1.1 ● PDSA Cycle

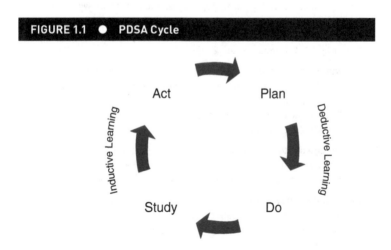

FIGURE 1.2 ● Three Broad Improvement Phases

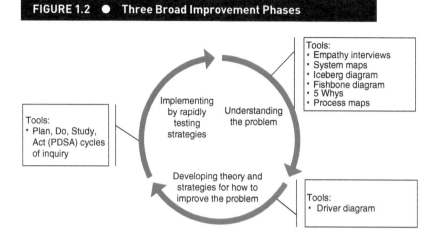

Understanding the Problem

Before attempting to improve or solve a problem, evaluators first need to identify and understand the cause (or causes) of the problem. We live in an action- and solution-oriented world. It is easy to impatiently jump right to the solution without taking the time to fully understand why there is problem. Others have referred to this phenomenon as "solutionitus" (Bryk et al., 2015). Root cause and causal systems analysis tools such as the 5 Whys protocol and the Cause and Effect diagram, also known as the *fishbone* or *Ishikawa diagram*, help teams dig deep or go wide across the system, thus preventing solutionitus. There are also other improvement tools that are often used in the phase, including empathy interviews, system maps, iceberg diagram, and process maps.

Developing a Theory for Improving the Problem

Evaluators are very familiar with the concept of a theory of change or a theory of action. Improvement science has an analogous tool, known as a *Driver Diagram* or *Theory of Improvement*. The tool, shown in Figure 1.3, has a similar purpose as a logic model but with more of system-wide focus. The system can be bounded in different ways to have a narrower or broader focus. In Figure 1.3, the system is bounded more narrowly to the classroom.[4] The aim, shown in the box on the far left, is the measurable goal. The Primary Drivers identify the high-leverage focal areas in the system that would drive the change in the aim. High-leverage refers to the idea of focusing on those areas within the system that will provide the "most bang for your buck." Using the information gained in the Understanding the Problem phase, a team considers what causes they can address with the fewest resources (or currently available resources) and will have the biggest impacts.

---

[4] The case study, presented in Part 2 of this book, provides details about the decision to narrowly focus this driver diagram.

FIGURE 1.3 ● Driver Diagram Example

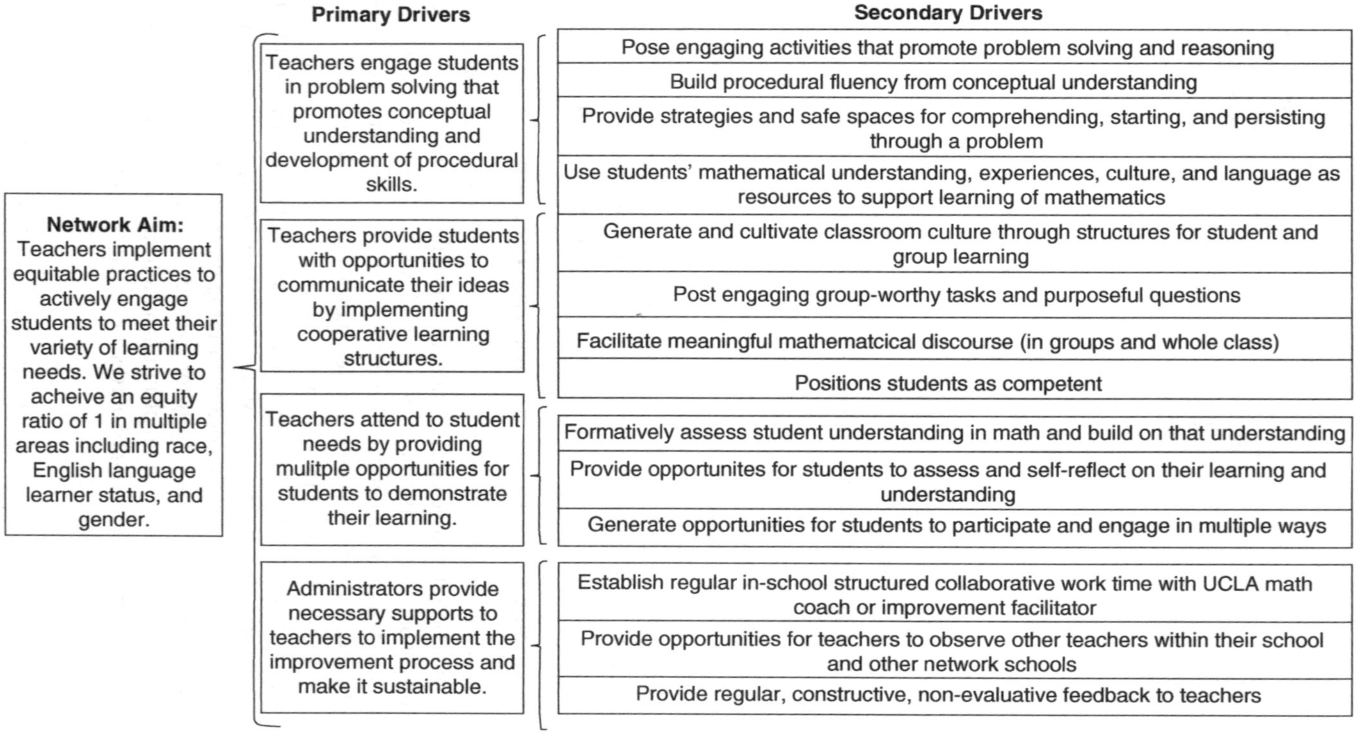

Network Aim:
Teachers implement equitable practices to actively engage students to meet their variety of learning needs. We strive to achieve an equity ratio of 1 in multiple areas including race, English language learner status, and gender.

Primary Drivers

Primary Driver	Secondary Drivers
Teachers engage students in problem solving that promotes conceptual understanding and development of procedural skills.	Pose engaging activities that promote problem solving and reasoning
	Build procedural fluency from conceptual understanding
	Provide strategies and safe spaces for comprehending, starting, and persisting through a problem
	Use students' mathematical understanding, experiences, culture, and language as resources to support learning of mathematics
Teachers provide students with opportunities to communicate their ideas by implementing cooperative learning structures.	Generate and cultivate classroom culture through structures for student and group learning
	Post engaging group-worthy tasks and purposeful questions
	Facilitate meaningful mathematical discourse (in groups and whole class)
	Positions students as competent
Teachers attend to student needs by providing multiple opportunities for students to demonstrate their learning.	Formatively assess student understanding in math and build on that understanding
	Provide opportunites for students to assess and self-reflect on their learning and understanding
	Generate opportunities for students to participate and engage in multiple ways
Administrators provide necessary supports to teachers to implement the improvement process and make it sustainable.	Establish regular in-school structured collaborative work time with UCLA math coach or improvement facilitator
	Provide opportunities for teachers to observe other teachers within their school and other network schools
	Provide regular, constructive, non-evaluative feedback to teachers

The Secondary Drivers unpack the broad Primary Drivers, thereby leading to more manageable and actionable steps. Change ideas—those strategies for improvement to be tested through the PDSA cycles—"plug in" to these secondary drivers; they should be developed to improve the secondary drivers. Notably, these are all hypothesized theories. Driver diagrams are dynamic and should always be updated with the most recent emergent learnings about a problem.

Implementing by Rapidly Testing Strategies and Generating New Knowledge

The PDSA is a format for rapidly testing potential strategies (change ideas) aligned with the drivers. Importantly, it is a vehicle for reflective practice. The prediction surfaces assumptions, what one expects to happen while implementing a change idea. Evidence is collected, and then the individual and/or team reflect on whether they met the assumption, and why or why not. With this new knowledge, the team can choose to scale up a change idea, adapt it and conduct another PDSA cycle, or abandon it all together. Ultimately, this knowledge provides more understanding around the problem, potentially altering the theory for how to improve it.

Although Deming's ideas were grounded in industry and manufacturing, they have expanded to other fields. Currently, improvement science is most prevalent in healthcare. Don Berwick, the founder of the Institute for Healthcare Improvement (IHI), was one of the early champions of improvement science. Improvement science has successfully cracked vexing healthcare challenges such as how to reduce the number of child asthma-related visits to the emergency room (C. E. Williams, 2015).

Improvement science has spread to education in recent years, as demonstrated by the aforementioned community college example. The Carnegie Foundation combined the improvement science model with the concept of networked improvement communities when they formed a network of practitioners and experts who collaboratively experimented with innovative common practices and consistent measures across the community colleges. K–12 schools are also embracing improvement science, as demonstrated by this book's case study.

Other Continuous Improvement Approaches

It should be noted that there are other improvement models. Below are brief descriptions. While not an exhaustive list, it does represent the more commonly known models in manufacturing, health care, and education.

Six Sigma: Six Sigma is another improvement science model focused on organizational quality improvement. The concepts behind it originated in the 1970s when an engineer at Motorola developed a new quality assurance methodology aimed at reducing process variation. The model incorporated

Walter Shewart's ideas around variation: Variation that fell outside of three standard deviations (sigma) from the mean, up or down, required a correction (Six Sigma Global Institute [SSGI], 2020). The goal was to improve consistency of processes, and thus, performance. Six Sigma practices can now be found in numerous and varying sectors, including manufacturing, retail corporations, government, and health care (American Society for Quality [ASQ], 2020a).

There are more specified models within the Six Sigma approach. The define, measure, analyze, improve, and control (DMAIC) is one of those. DMAIC is a data-driven quality improvement framework with the five phases representing the different stages of the process (ASQ, 2020a).

- Define the problem, improvement activity, project goals.

- Measure the process performance by developing process maps, capability analysis, and pareto charts.

- Analyze the process to determine root causes of problem or poor performance.

- Improve the process performance by addressing the root cause. May use approach where you rapidly introduce change, conduct controlled test, and apply statistical design of experiments (DOE) method.

- Control the improved process and future process performance by documenting and monitoring process behavior. The goal is to ensure process consistency within three sigma, up or down.

Lean: Lean is a set of management practices and techniques aimed at eliminating non-value-added activities, thereby, improving efficiency and effectiveness (ASQ, 2020b). Lean began in the automobile industry, dating back to Henry Ford's mass production intention of increasing efficiency (SSGI, 2020). Toyota is a well-known champion of the method. They have developed systems to reduce waste in processes and procedures so that all work adds value. Lean practices are also used in various sectors, including manufacturing, finance, and health care.

Lean Six Sigma: This approach combines ideas from Six Sigma and Lean to improve performance by improving consistency of process performance and increasing efficiency and reducing waste. Lean Six Sigma also incorporates the DMAIC model, with a broader focus on the problem rather than just on the process (SSGI, 2019) and can be found in use in numerous sectors, including government, health care, industry.

Data Wise: The Data Wise project developed out of the Harvard Graduate School of Education to support educators engaged in collaborative inquiry.

The aim of this model is to integrate data-driven inquiry into instruction and district improvement. Their Universal Data Wise Improvement Process includes the following steps (Lockwood et al., 2017):

- Organize for collaborative work by establishing structures and teams

- Build data literacy to increase comfort with data

- Create data overview to identify a focal question to address

- Dig into data to address the focal question and identify a learner-centered problem

- Examine own practice and identify a focal problem of practice

- Develop action plan

- Plan to assess progress

- Act and assess by implementing plan and gathering, reviewing, and reflecting upon evidence of improvement

Lesson Study: Lesson study is a cycle of inquiry process that originated in Japan as a collaboration among teachers to improve instruction. As such, it is a collaborative inquiry process whereby teachers plan a lesson with fellow teachers, collect data regarding the lesson, review and reflect on those data, and revise the lesson as needed. There are four broad steps (The Lesson Study Group at Mills College, 2018; Teacher Development Trust, 2015):

- Study: Teams of teachers collaborate to investigate a potential problem, review relevant research, and identify a goal for students.

- Plan: The teachers plan a lesson together that addresses the issue raised in the Study phase. They predict how students will react to the lesson and determine what student data to collect.

- Teach: One team member teaches the lesson, while the other teachers collect student data around student thinking and learning.

- Reflect: The team meets after the lesson to discuss the data, reflect on what they learned, and consider whether it met their prediction. They then decide how to revise the lesson.

Ultimately, all these approaches and models can be considered formative evaluation because they focus on improvement, be it a process, a problem, an organization, or a system, with the intention of enhancing knowledge and decision making (Russ-Eft & Preskill, 2009). Yet continuous improvement is a distinct form of formative evaluation because of its *continuous* nature. This feature lends itself to being a powerful vehicle for change. The evaluation team can uncover and address emergent needs by ongoing disciplined inquiry. Improving persistent problems requires agility and responsiveness. As the soup example has shown us, contextual conditions rarely remain static.

Conclusion

Improvement approaches fall under the broad umbrella of formative evaluation. The decision of which model to use will depend on your purpose, problem, and type of system in which you are situated. When attempting to improve a problem, diagnosing whether it exists in an organized system or complex system is a key first step (Rohanna & Christie, in preparation). Chapter 2 prepares the reader for this task by discussing the idea of systems and complexity in more depth, while Part 2 begins the case study of applying an improvement science framework within a complex system. By better understanding which approach to utilize, evaluators are better positioned in their quest for leading change.

Questions for Discussion

1. Why does the author consider improvement science to be an evaluative strategy for change?

2. What persistent problems have you encountered in your own settings or organizations?

3. How might improvement science or another continuous improvement model be applied to that problem?

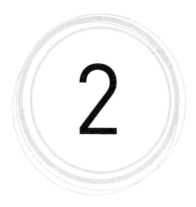

The Truth About Complex Systems

The idea of complex systems is nothing new. But while seemingly self-explanatory, these two words are actually a nebulous, abstract concept in evaluation, research, and improvement practice. For years, I thought I truly understood complex systems: A whole set has interrelated, dependent parts, and a change to one part results in a consequential change to another part. True. But effecting change within complex systems, especially where many of our persistent societal problems live, requires a deeper understanding of complexity science and systems thinking. This chapter continues our journey into leading change through evaluation by furthering our vital understanding of these ideas and illuminating the need for embracing the perspectives and experiences of actors within these systems.

In this chapter, I cover:

- Systems and Complexity Science
  - Complex Adaptive Systems
  - The Cynefin Framework
  - Causal Feedback Loops
- Learning Your Way Through Problems
- Multiple and Inclusive Perspectives: The Need for Embracing Actors Within the System
- Building Capacity for Participatory Approaches

Systems and Complexity Science

Donella Meadows (2008), one of the leading systems thinkers, defines a system as "an interconnected set of elements that is coherently organized in a way that achieves something" (p. 11). According to Meadows, a system "must consist of three kinds of things: *elements, interconnections,* and a *function* or *purpose*" (p. 11).

Systems also have espoused purposes: what the system is promoted as doing (e.g., providing a quality education to all students). And systems have actual purposes: what the system is actually producing due to its current design, whether intended or unintended (Stroh, 2015). Persistent problems often exist within complex systems when their actual system patterns are in conflict with their espoused purposes (Stroh, 2015).

As an example, we can consider a hospital. A hospital is a system with elements consisting of doctors, patients, medicine, operating rooms, and so on. These elements are interconnected through policies, procedures and administrations for the espoused system purpose of providing quality health care. Now consider the alarming statistic that pregnancy-related mortality rates for Black women are over three times that of their white counterparts (Petersen et al., 2019). There is a systemic inequity. Actual system patterns are in direct conflict with the espoused purpose of the hospital (Rohanna & Christie, in preparation).

EXAMPLE 2.1

EDUCATION SYSTEM IN CONFLICT WITH
ESPOUSED PURPOSE

K–12 education is another example of a complex system with serious conflicts with its espoused purpose. The K–12 system is composed of schools interconnected through curriculum and assessment policies and providers, federal policies such as Every Student Succeeds Act, and widespread structural and instructional norms on "how to teach." While the education system exists to provide a quality education and help all students succeed, the system does not consistently achieve its espoused purpose. This is particularly true for students of color and those designated as low-income. Again, a troubling, persistent, and systemic problem.

Note: Although more could be said about the education system and its history of systemic oppression as the reason for why the system is designed to achieve the results it does, this book assumes that many educators are working in the system today to improve these injustices yet struggle with their goals because of the complexity of the system.

To diagnose, understand, and improve persistent problems within complex systems, we must first have a deeper understanding of complexity and system dynamics. There are various frameworks for conceptualizing why problems persevere in complex systems. In this chapter, I describe three.

Complex Adaptive Systems

Complex Adaptive Systems is a complexity theory based on the work of Ralph Stacey (1996) and Brenda Zimmerman et al. (1998) that considers social systems on a range of two factors: agreement and certainty. Agreement refers to agreement among individuals in groups, teams, and organizations about their priorities and the activities in which they engage. Certainty refers to the cause and effect predictability of relationships among actions, conditions, and consequences (Parsons, 2012; Stacey, 1996; Zimmerman et al., 1998; Zimmerman & Dooley, 2001). System dynamics can be categorized around the degrees of agreement and certainty (Figure 2.1). System dynamics refers to emergent and changing interactions among elements within a system(s) (American Evaluation Association Systems in Evaluation Topical Interest Group, 2018). In this framework, they can be described as one of three types: organized, adaptive (self-organizing), and unorganized.

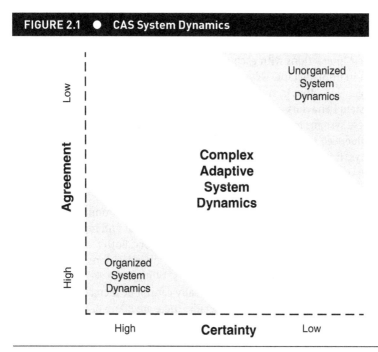

FIGURE 2.1 ● CAS System Dynamics

Source: Adapted from Parsons, B. (2012). Using Complexity Science Concepts When Designing System Interventions and Evaluations. http://insites.org/resource/using-complexity-science-concepts-when-designing-system-interventions-and-evaluations/

- **Organized System Dynamics:** When the degrees of agreement and certainty are high, the system dynamics tend to be stable, organized, and predictable. Organizations such as manufacturers are very structured with hierarchical chains of command and can assume this type of system dynamic. For example, an increase in labor hours—assuming the workers are in accord—may reliably result in an increase in production.[1]

  Evaluations and research that predict a linear cause and effect relationship of an action to an outcome implicitly (or explicitly) make the assumption of operating within organized system dynamics. For example, in some hierarchical structures such as schools, it may be expected that there is high agreement among administrators, teachers, and parents in implementing interventions to help student learning and the assumption that providing an intervention, if it is effective, will lead to an improved student outcome (effective intervention -> improved student outcome). However, these assumptions may not always hold true, particularly if the system dynamics lean toward self-organizing rather than organized.

- **Complex Adaptive System Dynamics:** Between organized and unorganized system dynamics falls adaptive system dynamics, also referred to as *self-organizing and complex adaptive systems* (CAS) (i.e., a complex system). In a system with this dynamic, there are many semi-independent and diverse agents who continually adapt to their interactions with each other and their environment and may act in unpredictable ways (Parsons, 2012). While not completely organized—that is, not a high degree of agreement or certainty to the system behaviors—system patterns do exist. Furthermore, control in these systems is distributive rather than centralized. Agents can be influenced rather than directly ordered to follow or behave in certain ways. It is through identifying high leverage areas for influence that self-organization dynamics can be understood and leveraged to effect positive change (Parsons, 2012).

  Organizations where there is structure, but also autonomy of its diverse actors, may assume this system dynamic. Schools and hospitals, although structured, may fall into this category. Both teachers and doctors have the autonomy to make their own decisions based on their interactions with system elements. While there are policies and processes in place, their actions usually cannot be dictated. They can, however, be influenced. Additionally, there are many diverse agents in education and health care systems.

---

[1] That is, it could be expected to increase up to a certain point based on the economic law of diminishing returns.

- **Unorganized System Dynamics:** At the other end of the spectrum, where the degrees of agreement and certainty are low, the system dynamics tend to be random and disorganized. Systems have basically collapsed actions, and events are unpredictable and seem disconnected with no discernable patterns (Parsons, 2012). Hurricane Maria, which devastated Puerto Rico in September 2017, is an example of unorganized system dynamics. The event and aftermath were seemingly chaotic because the storm damaged cell towers, roads, an already precarious electrical grid due to the recent Hurricane Irma, and more. Low agreement among key actors, such as the White House administration, Puerto's Rico's administrative officials, and the Federal Emergency Management Agency about priorities and necessary actions contributed to the instability of the event.

The Cynefin Framework

The Cynefin Framework is a sense-making framework to help leaders make decisions when faced with complexity. Developed by Snowden, Boone, and Kurtz, it incorporates complexity science and organizational theory (Kurtz & Snowden, 2003; Snowden & Boone, 2007). Their use of the Welsh word "Cynefin" (pronounced ku-nev-in) recognizes that "all human interactions are strongly influenced and frequently determined by the patterns of our multiple experiences" (Kurtz & Snowden, 2003, p. 467). They posit that the assumptions of order, rational choice, and intentional capability (i.e., actions by others are deliberate) do not hold true in all contexts even though many tools and strategies assume they do. There are five delineated contexts in which to make sense of situations and act accordingly: simple, complicated, complex, chaotic, and disorder. These categories are codified by predictive abilities, the character of the relationship between cause and effect.

- **Simple:** Simple contexts tend to be stable, with clear cause and effect relationships among elements. In this context, managing situations is straightforward and the answer is usually apparent. Leaders must sense, categorize, and respond to situations, potentially drawing on similar past experiences or best practices. This is the realm of the "known knowns" (Snowden & Boone., 2007, p. 2). This categorization is similar to organized system dynamics in CAS theory. A machine breaks down in a manufacturing plant. The shift manager (i.e., leader) calls the plant's mechanic to fix it.

- **Complicated:** Complicated contexts also tend to have cause and effect relationships; however, these relationships may not be fully known or apparent to everyone. There also may be multiple correct and knowable options that a leader can take to address a situation. A leader in this context must sense and analyze (rather than simply categorize) to respond to situations and may often need to seek expert guidance. This is the realm of the "known unknowns" (Snowden & Boone,, 2007, p. 3). An automotive executive wants to improve diminishing sales of a prevalent car and seeks experts in the company to develop a new fresh model. While the change could predictability boost sales, the market's preference may be unclear. The situation requires analysis and innovation.

- **Complex:** Like Complex Adaptive Systems, complex contexts in the Cynefin Framework are characterized by unpredictability, no apparent cause and effect relationships, and emergent patterns. The context is interdependent: A change in one place can result in a change in another (i.e., interconnections among elements). Patterns cannot be predicted but they can be understood, and importantly, understood from multiple perspectives. Rather than trying to impose best practices or known solutions, a leader in a complex context should provide the safe space for the best course of action to emerge and conduct experiments to learn. Snowden and Boone (2007) provide an example to illustrate this idea:

> There is a scene in the film *Apollo 13* when the astronauts encounter a crisis ("Houston, we have a problem") that moves the situation into a complex domain. A group of experts is put in a room with a mismatch of materials—bits of plastic and odds and ends that mirror the resources available to the astronauts in flight. Leaders tell the team: This is what you have; find a solution or the astronauts will die. None of those experts knew a priori what would work. Instead, they had to let a solution emerge from the materials at hand. And they succeeded. (p. 5)

- **Chaotic:** In chaotic contexts, cause and effect relationships are unknowable because they are constantly shifting. Patterns cannot be identified, and thus, cannot be leveraged or managed. This is the realm of the "unknowables." With no known right answer, leaders must act swiftly and decisively, because most of these situations arise due to a crisis. Snowden and Boone use the events of 9/11 as an example of a situation that falls into this context (Snowden & Boone., 2007, p. 5).

- **Disorder:** The fifth category of disorder applies only when the other four contexts cannot be discerned. The Cynefin Framework does not provide guidance for leadership actions in this state.

Causal Feedback Loops

Causal feedback loops are components of system dynamics modeling. System dynamics modeling was developed by Jay Forrester and other scholars at Massachusetts Institute Technology in the late 1950s. System dynamics modeling provides a framework for understanding system patterns, including feedback mechanisms and system pressures. These feedback mechanisms and underlying pressures shape a system's behavior—think of vicious or virtuous cycles—and thus, give insight into a system's actual purpose versus its espoused purpose.

Because systems dynamics modeling including stocks and flows and in-depth computer simulations built from diverse data representing numerous variables encompasses more than is discussed in this chapter, I have chosen instead to refer to the framework discussed here as *causal feedback loop diagrams*.

Causal feedback loop diagrams equate the same ideas but in a more practical way that can be implemented by those not familiar with computer simulation modeling. Rather, the tools of causal feedback loops can be applied with a pen, paper, and a knowledgeable team using continuous improvement cycles of inquiry.

Peter Senge (2006) introduced the idea of causal feedback loop diagramming to a more mainstream public with his book *The Fifth Discipline*. In his book, he discussed the five disciplines necessary for a learning organization. He referred to the fifth discipline—systems thinking—as the cornerstone of a learning organization.[2] Systems thinking refers to the ability to see the whole rather than the parts (interconnections) and for understanding how underlying structures and pressures drive a system's behavior.

"Every system is perfectly designed to get the results it gets."[3] Causal loop diagramming is a tool for understanding how a system is designed, whether intentionally or unintentionally, to lead to certain outcomes. Thus, rather than a theory primarily about understanding complexity like Complex Adaptive Systems or the Cynefin Framework, causal loop diagramming is a strategy for addressing complexity. As such, this chapter devotes more space to its description.

David Peter Stroh (2015), a colleague of Senge's, uses the parable of the blind men and the elephant to explain systems thinking. In the parable, there are six blind men who are curious about elephants, a great beast they had often heard about but obviously never seen. One day, an elephant came to their village. They sought it out to learn more about it. The first blind man touched the side of the elephant and exclaimed, "It is like a wall." The second man touched the tusk. "It is strong and smooth," he said. The third, who touched the trunk, claimed, "It is like a snake." The fourth touched the elephant's legs and declared, "It is like a tree." The fifth man touched the elephant's ears and said, "It is like a fan." Last, the sixth man felt the elephant's tail and noted,

---

[2] The other four disciplines are continually working toward personal mastery, understanding and working with mental models, building a shared vision, and team learning.

[3] While this quote has been attributed to different authors over the years, it was most likely first stated by Paul Batalden from the Institute for Healthcare Improvement. More information can be found at http://www.ihi.org/communities/blogs/origin-of-every-system-is-perfectly-designed-quote.

FIGURE 2.2 ● **Blind Men and the Elephant**

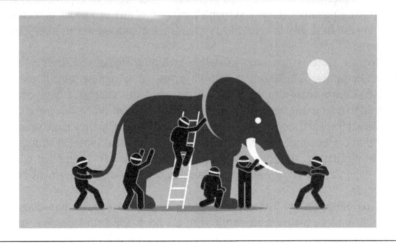

iStock.com/leremy

"It is like a rope." Not understanding why each of them had such different perceptions, they began arguing with each other, each claiming that they were correct. A wise man who was passing by heard them arguing. He stopped and told that they were all correct. The blind men were shocked and did not understand how that was possible. The wise man stated that they each touched a different part of the elephant and the whole elephant consisted of all those different traits.

Like the blind men, many of us work in organizations and systems where we may not initially see the whole. Instead, we tend to see the part that is in front of us and may struggle with another's perspective because it does not represent our own. Systems thinking is a way to see the whole elephant.

This parable highlights one of three valuable concepts necessary for systems thinking: multiple perspectives (Williams & Iman, 2007). People can have different views about the same system, and the same problem. Interrelationships, which we have already touched on, and boundaries are the other two concepts (Williams & Iman, 2007). To improve a problem within a large complex system, it needs to be bounded. It is not possible to address all parts of the system at once. The concept of boundaries not only refers to time and space, but also to which stakeholders are included in understanding the system. As the Newark Public School example discussed later in this chapter illustrates, those hoping to lead change need to seriously consider whose voices are being privileged and whose are being marginalized in the systems analysis (Midgley, 2007; B. Williams, 2015). Systems thinking should be inclusive.

Therefore, as an essential tool for systems thinking, those engaging in causal loop diagramming need to embrace multiple perspectives to understand system dynamics and interconnected elements, create space for sometimes marginalized voices, and bound the system to the problem they are trying to solve. Trying to diagram causal feedback loops for a whole system could be overwhelming, and potentially too macro for identifying levers of change. Rather, one should start first with the problem and bound the system and causal feedback loop to it.

Senge (2006) refers to two types of causal feedback loops—reinforcing and balancing—as the "building blocks" of systems thinking (p. 79). In the systems thinking context, the term *feedback* does not have its typical meaning when we think about improvement: providing information or input about someone's performance, product, act, and so on. In this case, feedback refers to the idea that cyclical patterns result when a system(s) *feeds on itself*. The system's elements and interconnections are driving the system's dynamics, which importantly, may or may not be the system's espoused purpose.

Reinforcing Feedback Loops

A system demonstrating reinforcing feedback loops accelerates its rate growth or decline exponentially toward some outcome. Depending on the situation, this can create a virtuous (positive) cycle or a vicious (negative) cycle. An example of how a reinforcing feedback loop can create a vicious cycle can be found in toilet paper.

At the beginning of the COVID-19 pandemic, fearful people began stockpiling toilet paper. This caused others who did not initially fear running out of toilet paper to rush out and buy up toilet paper, too. Toilet paper manufacturers were not prepared for this sudden demand. As a result, stores actually did run

FIGURE 2.3 ● Toilet Paper Reinforcing Feedback Loop

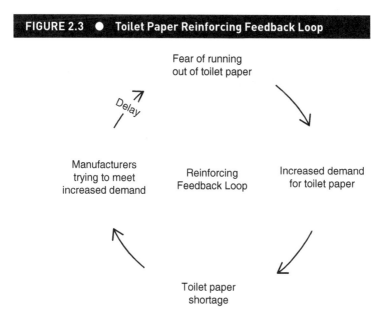

out of toilet paper. Had everyone stuck to their usual buying habits, there likely would have been enough toilet paper for everyone. This vicious cycle could only be broken by disrupting the pattern. Retailers imposed strict limits on the amount of toilet paper one could buy in a single purchase, thus allowing more shoppers to buy toilet paper during the delay when manufacturers were working hard to step up production of toilet paper and for stores to restock their shelves.

Balancing Feedback Loops

A system is stuck in the status quo when demonstrating a balancing cycle. This can be a positive if the goal is to stabilize a system, or a negative if the goal is to improve an outcome but nothing seems to change despite numerous initiatives. Balancing feedback loops are common in education systems that are striving to improve and respond to a target outcome. Figure 2.4 provides an example of this. The Smarter Balance summative assessment provides data around the percentage of students who perform at grade level in math and English Language Arts. Often in the cases where a large percentage of students do not perform at grade level, school district officials will put pressure on school administrators (e.g., principals) to meet a set target, as shown in Figure 2.4. In response, school district and school administrators may institute a new intervention and put pressure on teachers to quickly implement it. If they review the assessment results again (usually at the beginning of the next school year) and find they did not meet the target, they may deem the intervention ineffective and abandon it for a new intervention. In reality, there is often a delay before seeing improvement. This *adopt, attack, abandon* cycle is a detrimental pattern that can continue indefinitely, resulting in assessment scores hovering around the same percentage year-to-year.

Therefore, and ironically, implementing such a data-driven process, where the primary tasks are to gather outcome data and hold educators accountable,

---

FIGURE 2.4 ● Adopt, Attack, Abandon Balancing Feedback Loop

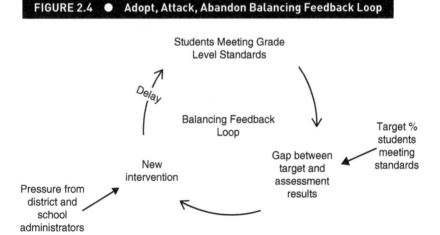

Students Meeting Grade Level Standards

Delay

Balancing Feedback Loop

Target % students meeting standards

New intervention

Gap between target and assessment results

Pressure from district and school administrators

can result in the system being stuck in a balancing feedback loop. One reason is the concept of delays, a *normal part of any system*. However, many actors in systems, particularly those who hold others accountable, intentionally or unintentionally ignore the reality of the lag between implementation and results. Instead, they may hold a belief or assumption that change should be immediately apparent, or that others are resisting change or just not trying hard enough.

While the idea of mapping causal feedback loops seems daunting, there are many patterns common to numerous social systems. These are called *system archetypes*. Some prevalent ones are shown in Example 2.2, but there are many more. Understanding these archetypes can be very helpful for diagnosing, responding, and changing non-beneficial causal feedback patterns. More information about these archetypes can be found in Senge's and David Peter Stroh's writings (Senge, 2006; Senge et al., 1994; Stroh, 2015).

EXAMPLE 2.2
COMMON SYSTEM ARCHETYPES IN EDUCATION

Fixes That Fail: This system pattern represents the idea of implementing a quick solution to fix an immediate problem, but in actuality it leads to unexpected long-term consequences that hinder the desired improvement. A real-world example would be the aforementioned (Chapter 1) California community colleges move to require many incoming students to take remedial math courses in preparation for college-level courses. This "fix" resulted in the long-term consequence of some students dropping out rather than succeeding because taking more math classes created more opportunities to fail a course.

Shifting the Burden: This is another common system pattern that occurs when the burden of a problem is shifted to other issues or people. In education, an example of shifting the burden was the popular notion that students were to blame for low math grades and assessment scores rather than a need for reevaluating instructional practices. This trend suggested that many students did not have a *growth mindset* or a belief that they could develop their math abilities, and this was why they did not learn math. Unfortunately, this idea became so popular that many educators focused on student effort and motivation to persist, with less attention paid to whether students were being taught the tools and strategies to solve a math problem in the first place.

Accidental Adversaries: Ironically, this system pattern can result when there are too many good intentions and too many providers who want to help. There are so many outside helpers (e.g., university, foundations) who are advocating and supporting initiatives to help students, they begin to compete for teachers' time and attention. Nonprofits may also struggle with the accidental adversaries system when numerous funders push programs and interventions that result in too many endeavors, essentially competing against each other for time and resources.

Understanding system patterns requires using systems thinking tools such as causal feedback loops, system archetypes, driver diagrams, and actor maps, to name a few. By using these tools, evaluators can begin to understand the levers for systems change. For example, with accidental adversaries, one would consider how to improve the communication with outside funders and facilitate systemic conversations so everyone can see the role they play. What programs or initiatives might they give up to support the greater system goal (Stroh, 2015)?

Learning Your Way Through Problems

In complex systems, the notions of predictability and linear thinking are thrown out the window and replaced by nonlinearity, unpredictability, emergence, and system patterns. These concepts can be challenging in evaluation, where causal links tend to be conceptualized as flowing in one direction, linear, and predictive (think logic model). Thus, there may be an implicit assumption of operating within an organized system in many evaluations (Rohanna & Christie, in preparation).

All three of these frameworks suggest that our usual evaluation modus operandi may not fit this relatively new understanding of the paradigm of complexity. It is imperative for evaluators who are seeking to lead change to gain an understanding of complex system dynamics. The American Evaluation Association Systems in Evaluation Topical Interest Group (AEA SETIG) identifies systems evaluation principles that connect to the systems and complexity ideas already discussed. These principals can be found on their website and are organized around the concepts of interrelationships, perspectives, boundaries, and dynamics.[4]

Ideally, evaluators could use the complexity science and systems thinking ideas posited in this book, which connect to the SETIG principles, to understand how to diagnose, respond to and reset system patterns, and how to engage methods for utilizing and responding to emergence. Continuous improvement grounded in improvement science is one approach that evaluators can adopt for working with these concepts, particularly when considering complex systems' traits of unpredictability and emergence.

Let's return to the Apollo 13 example. In April 1970, Apollo 13 was on its way to the moon. Just 2 days into the mission, an oxygen tank exploded, putting the astronauts' lives in grave jeopardy. NASA leapt into action. Mission Control Flight Director Gene Kranz announced to his controllers, "Let's solve the problem, but let's not make it any worse by guessing" (Cass, 2005, Part 1 p. 5). In the 1995 film, *Apollo 13*, the crisis spawned two of the most famous movie quotes of all time: "Houston, we have a problem," and "Failure is not an

---

[4]https://www.systemsinevaluation.com/wp-content/uploads/2018/10/SETIG-Principles-FINAL-DRAFT-2018-9-9.pdf

option."[5] Even if you've never seen the film, you know the lines because they now live in the American vernacular.

In reality, NASA crews were prepared to solve emerging complex problems because they had cultivated a culture of continuous improvement, as told by Stephen Cass (2005) in a series of articles titled *Apollo 13, We Have a Solution.*

When the oxygen tank exploded, the three astronauts needed to temporarily move from their damaged three-man command service module (CSM) into the landing module (LM), which was designed for two people. But there was a problem. The LM's power was off to conserve energy. Switching it on required power from the CSM, but it had lost fuel cells in the explosion and could no longer supply it. The astronauts were running out of oxygen and could not move into the LM until the power was turned on. They needed a solution, and fast.

One year earlier, Apollo 10 preflight simulations created the crisis that was now happening on Apollo 13. Apollo 10's fuel cells had failed in simulation at *almost the exact spot* they had just failed on Apollo 13.

In the Apollo 10 simulation, the crew died. Some at NASA dismissed the results. They thought the simulation was unrealistic: It required too many complex system failures to occur on both modules for it to result in actual deaths.

Luckily, the lunar module branch chief could not dismiss the simulated outcome. Over the next few months, his team ran simulation after simulation and developed solutions for multiple scenarios. Their results had not yet been officially certified by the time Apollo 13 launched. Now, they needed to pull those results "off the shelf." The team was able to move the Apollo 13 crew into the LM with only 15 minutes to spare. Continuous improvement thinking had saved the astronauts' lives.

They succeeded because rather than dismissing a previous failure they chose to learn from it. The simulations gave them the safe space and the time to learn and experiment, thereby allowing them to learn from each new unpredictable and emergent problem.

While many of society's complex problems are not the stuff of movies, they are just as important. The case study in this book, albeit less dramatic, also illustrates how professionals with diverse expertise collaborated using continuous improvement methods to first diagnose and understand the problem they were trying to solve—the high percentage of students failing math courses—and learn their way through the problem, using an iterative process for testing new solutions and responding to emergent challenges. However, methods alone are not enough. Like the story of the Apollo 13, potential solutions require the expertise and experience of those who are closest to the problem.

---

[5] In actuality, Kranz never spoke those words. However, he did give an inspiring speech to his controllers to bolster their confidence that they would successfully bring the crew home. Cass, S. (2005). *Apollo 13, We Have a Solution* (Part 2). https://spectrum.ieee.org/tech-history/space-age/apollo-13-we-have-a-solution-part-2

Multiple and Inclusive Perspectives: The Need for Embracing Actors Within the System

One December night in 2009, Newark, New Jersey, Mayor Cory Booker and Governor-elect Chris Christie toured the dangerous streets of New Jersey's most populated city. As described by Dale Russakoff's *The New Yorker* article and her 2015 book, *The Prize*, Booker had invited Christie to join him on a late-night ride to learn about his crime-fighting efforts. During that tour, the two discussed the state of Newark's public schools; Booker's real motivation for extending the invitation.

Booker was an advocate of charter schools, and Christie had recently raised the issue of urban schools in his gubernatorial campaign. That night, the two made a pact to reform Newark's schools. Booker's own words best sum up the nature of that pact: "We have to grab this system by the roots and yank it out and start over. It's outrageous" (Russakoff, 2014, p. 58).

Booker's outrage was understandable. At the time, most Newark public school students were unable to read or do math at grade-level. Almost half were dropping out (Kotlowitz, 2015). School buildings were old and dilapidated. Its system of patronage jobs created a ratio of administrators and bureaucratic clerks to students that far exceeded the state's average yet did not result in better performance (Russakoff, 2014). When Booker was elected mayor of Newark in 2006, he encouraged the charter school movement. As a result, many parents pulled their children from the district, enrolled them in charter schools, and left the school district to serve students who tended to be the most economically and academically vulnerable.

Enter Mark Zuckerberg, the founder of Facebook. He was a 26-year-old billionaire, budding philanthropist, and, with his wife Priscilla Chan, searching for an education cause. In her book, Russakoff details how Booker won over Zuckerberg and enlisted him in his new initiative. The two, along with Christie, appeared on *The Oprah Winfrey Show*, where Zuckerberg announced he had pledged one hundred million dollars to Newark Public Schools, over 5 years. The audience leapt to a standing ovation. Excitement was in the air. People were hopeful for *real* transformative change. One hundred million dollars, matched by millions more, could bring about a lot of positive change.

Four years later, most of the one hundred million dollars was spent. The outside experts, consultants, and reformers had left town. The school superintendent was gone. And nothing had changed. What went wrong?

Foretelling of mistakes to come, the famous day when Oprah Winfrey's audience heard about the Zuckerberg pledge was also the same day that Newark's parents and teachers heard about it for the first time, too (Russakoff, 2014).

From the beginning, the efforts were dominated by the perspectives of well-to-do and outside reformers. A new board called the Foundation for Newark's Future was formed, composed of donors who contributed five million dollars or more (Russakoff, 2014). By the time these donors formed a community advisory board (2 years later) most of the money was already committed to outside consultants, new labor contracts, and efforts to expand charter schools (Russakoff, 2014). Despite that fact that Newark residents expressed a desire to be involved at early community engagement forums, the voices of connected, expensive, consultants who were not familiar with Newark were privileged over theirs.

Christopher Serf, the former chief deputy to the New York Schools Chancellor, and Booker's informal education advisor, created a consulting firm specifically for the Newark project. He considered system reform to be his specialty and pronounced, "I'm very firmly of the view that when a system is a broken as this one you cannot fix it by doing the same things you've always done, only better" (Russakoff, 2014, p. 67). His solution was not to rethink the system. It was to dismantle it. Serf's firm led the charge to close and consolidate schools that were deemed low-performing in favor of charter schools. Unfortunately, that left the Newark public school system and its remaining students even worse off than before.

While Russakoff's account shares many more remarkable and important details, part of the story can be summed up by the fact that outside reformers favored shifting public money to charter schools, thereby depleting resources for public schools. Their actions revealed a lack of understanding of systems thinking, while they seemed to expect better performance by a system they were actually depleting. Furthermore, because the perspectives and voices of Newark's real stakeholders—teachers, principals, and parents—were dismissed, reformers missed the opportunity to see the whole system. Reform was done *to* stakeholders rather than *with* them. And it didn't work.

Building Capacity for Participatory Approaches

As we've now seen, systems change requires an understanding of system dynamics, systems thinking, and a willingness to value the perspectives of everyone in the system. In complex systems, people are semi-independent and diverse agents who continually adapt and act in unpredictable ways (Parsons, 2012). System stakeholders are an integral part of systems change. Thus, improving problems in complex systems requires a participatory and inclusive approach.

Participatory evaluators recognized this need a long time ago. In Participatory Evaluation (PE) evaluators collaborate with a program's primary users: those who are responsible for implementing the program or are closely connected the program (Alkin, 1991; Cousins, 2003; Cousins & Earl, 1992). PE engages primary users in the actual evaluation activities, including data collection, analysis, and interpretation of results (Cousins & Earl, 1992). By doing so, PE recognizes that knowledge is socially constructed (Cousins & Earl, 1992) and intends to foster the use of evaluation results by those most positioned to make changes or improvements.

Another participatory approach, Evaluative Inquiry, also acknowledges that inquiry is a "social and communal activity in which critical organizational issues are constructed by varied and broadly based community of inquirers"

(Preskill & Torres, 1999, p. 2). Similarly, improvement science, which is also participatory, seeks to combine the experiences and knowledge of frontline practitioners with those who hold the knowledge of how to improve (profound knowledge), who in the evaluation context, would be the evaluator (Christie et al., 2017; Rohanna, in press).

Paradoxically, the strength of participatory approaches is also one of its challenges. Authentically engaging *frontline workers* or primary users in inquiry requires they have the technical knowledge and capacity to apply the evaluative inquiry or improvement activities.

Fortunately, evaluators charged with leading change and building capacity in participatory frameworks can turn to evaluation capacity building sources for guidance. Though there are several similar definitions, evaluation capacity building can be succinctly defined as "an intentional process to increase individual motivation, knowledge, and skills, and to enhance a group or organization's ability to conduct or use evaluation" (Labin et al., 2012, p. 308).

Preskill and Boyle (2008) conceptualized a multidisciplinary model to guide practitioners in developing evaluation capacity. Their model drew on the fields of evaluation, organizational learning and change, and adult and workplace learning theories. Their model is shown in Figure 2.5.

First, the model designates the goal of evaluation capacity building as the development of evaluation knowledge, skills, and attitudes. It further acknowledges that those who initiate evaluation capacity building activities have various motivations, assumptions, and expectations regarding what they hope to achieve. Depending on these and the intended objective, there are 10 different evaluation teaching and learning strategies that can be employed:

1. Internship

2. Written Materials

3. Technology

4. Meetings

5. Appreciative Inquiry

6. Communities of Practice

7. Training

8. Involvement in Evaluation

9. Technical Assistance

10. Coaching

According to Preskill and Boyle's model, the learning needs to be transferred to the work context for this individual capacity to be sustained. Their model further deconstructs the processes, practices, policies, and resources required

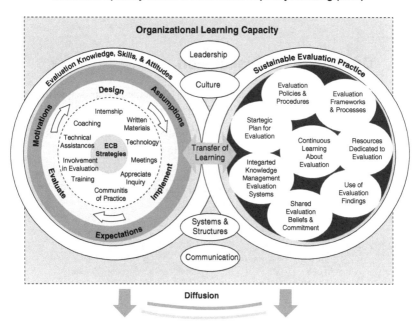

FIGURE 2.5 ● Preskill & Boyle's Multidisciplinary Evaluation Capacity Building Model

A Multidisciplinary Model of Evaluation Capacity Building (ECB)

for sustainable evaluation practice. Examples of these include the use of evaluation findings, integrated knowledge management evaluation system, continuous learning about evaluation, and so forth.

Accordingly, organizational capacity envelops teaching and learning strategies and sustainable evaluation practices. Preskill and Boyle posit that four areas of organizational capacity will influence the extent to which individuals will learn and build evaluation capacity and the extent to which it will be sustained. These four areas are: leadership, culture, systems & structures, and communication.

Conclusion

Solving persistent problems requires an understanding of complex system dynamics and systems thinking, which necessitates inclusiveness and multiple perspectives. Those closest to the problem may also have the greatest understanding of it. Preskill and Boyle's model provides a framework that evaluators can use when building the necessary capacity for participatory approaches and truly engaging participants in evaluative and improvement activities. Their model directed my own efforts for building the improvement science capacity of teachers featured in this book's case study. The beginning of Part 2 introduces the case study and explains how their model was at the heart of the study's conceptual framework.

Questions for Discussion

1. What type of system dynamics do you encounter in your own settings or organizations?

2. Why is it important to understand the dynamics of the system before attempting to improve a problem within it?

3. In the case of Newark Public Schools, what could reformers have done differently to more effectively foster change?

The Case Study

Introducing the Case Study

This book's case study examined one newly established improvement network founded by a large public university in Southern California, hereinafter called the University. It investigated the challenge of fully embracing and honoring the experiences and knowledge of frontline workers, in this case middle and high school math teachers, in effort to solve a persistent problem, high failure rates in math, while also charging them with implementing a technically demanding improvement science framework to improve that problem.

Adding to this conundrum was the fact that the University convened these teachers from five distinct schools as part of a networked improvement community. In the context of education, networked improvement communities are *inter*-organizational networks, whereby multiple schools join forces to tackle complex challenges. Networked improvement communities are a type of improvement science. Schools unite around improving one common problem of practice, such as high failure rates in math courses. They jointly dig deeper into the problem by sharing a diversity of experiences and then develop a plan for how to improve it. Teachers and administrators provide the practitioner experience and content knowledge, while specialists, typically from universities or other research institutions, share research-related content (e.g., math instruction expertise) and facilitate an improvement science framework for engaging in systematic inquiry.

The network hub's initial role is to lead the network in defining the shared problem of practice, and in more deeply analyzing the problem through root cause and causal systems analyses. Once these are established, the network hub directs the development of a theory of change framework for improving practices, which guides the work, also known as a *theory of improvement* or *driver diagram*.

Individual schools test this theory in practice, which typically involves multiple teachers experimenting with potential solutions in their classrooms. Through this process, educators within one school ideally form their own intra-organizational improvement community, where they share, learn, and generate new knowledge on a smaller scale than the network. These within-school learnings are then shared with all the other schools during periodic network gatherings. Multiple, varied new insights or knowledge from each school are integrated to continually inform the theory of practice improvement.

The Challenge

Networked improvement communities provide a promising approach for solving persistent problems in education. They utilize a continuous improvement framework grounded in improvement science, embrace variation that may occur across differing contexts, and engage both practitioners who are closest to the problem along with outside experts. However, the promising feature that embraces practitioner experience and knowledge can also create a challenge when considering the capacity needs of those engaging in the improvement activities. Networks who apply an improvement science framework require teachers and administrators to learn and apply technical methods related to causal systems analysis, theories of change, disciplined inquiry, and data collection and analysis. Learning how to engage in these technical activities can place an extra burden on teachers and administrators, which may be daunting and/or unrealistic given their existing duties. However, the network's ability to achieve success and solve complex problems of practice likely hinges on its ability to build improvement science capacity because knowledge is primarily generated through these improvement science tools. Without this crucial capacity, teachers and administrators may become frustrated when participating in these time-intensive network activities, with little improvement shown for their effort.

As such, the primary purposes of this case study were to examine how schools were prepared to successfully participate in the network and explain what facilitated successful participation. Successful implementation of improvement science was defined as a school's ability to execute Plan, Do, Study, Act (PDSA) cycles that were aligned with the driver diagram during Year 1 of the network. (Chapter 1 provides more explanation of PDSAs and the improvement science framework.)

Case Study Conceptual Framework

Figure P2.1 depicts the conceptual framework that guided this book's case study. It is grounded in Preskill and Boyle's (2008) multidisciplinary capacity building framework discussed in the previous chapter. This framework supported the development of the data collection instruments and protocols, along with my analysis. At the individual level, the network hub should

FIGURE P2.1 ● Case Study Conceptual Framework

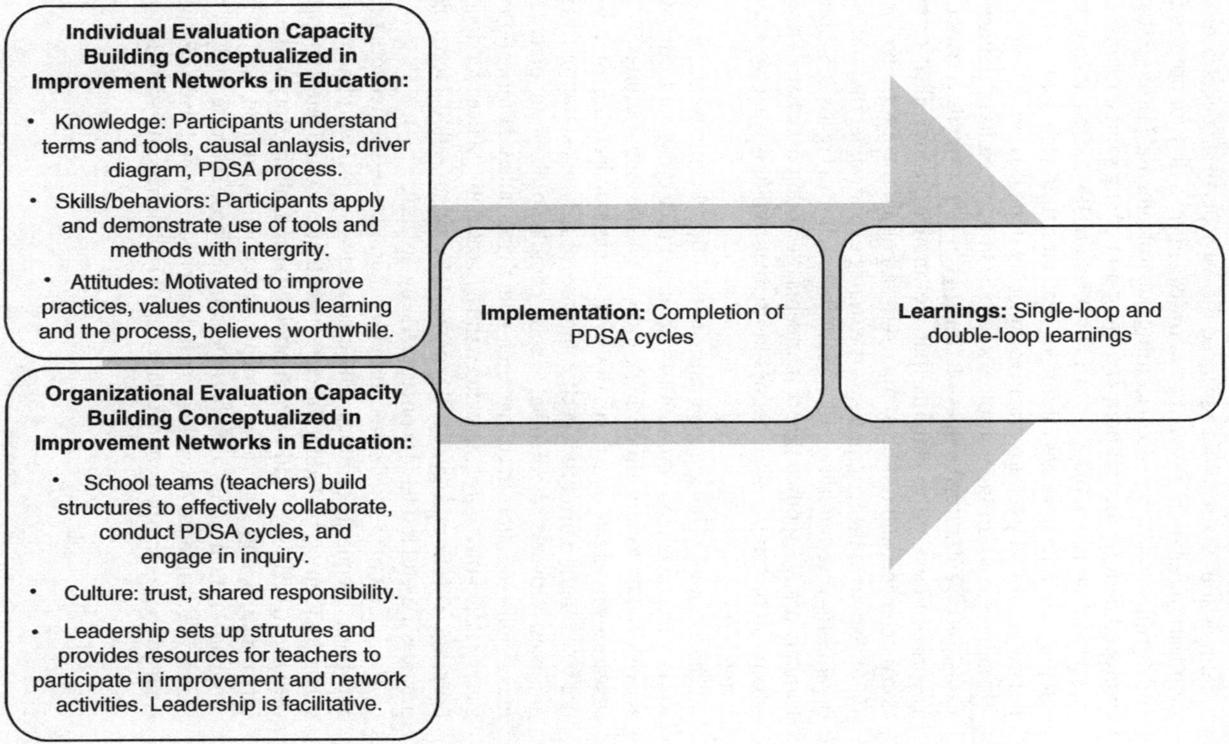

Individual Evaluation Capacity Building Conceptualized in Improvement Networks in Education:

- Knowledge: Participants understand terms and tools, causal anlaysis, driver diagram, PDSA process.

- Skills/behaviors: Participants apply and demonstrate use of tools and methods with intergrity.

- Attitudes: Motivated to improve practices, values continuous learning and the process, believes worthwhile.

Organizational Evaluation Capacity Building Conceptualized in Improvement Networks in Education:

- School teams (teachers) build structures to effectively collaborate, conduct PDSA cycles, and engage in inquiry.

- Culture: trust, shared responsibility.

- Leadership sets up structures and provides resources for teachers to participate in improvement and network activities. Leadership is facilitative.

Implementation: Completion of PDSA cycles

Learnings: Single-loop and double-loop learnings

consider capacity related to knowledge, skills/behaviors, and attitudes. At the organizational level, schools need to embed collaborative structures and the network hub should attend to the culture and leadership support. The framework further suggests that building teacher and school capacity in these areas will contribute to the implementation of PDSA cycles, which will then lead to network learnings. I further conceptualized these learnings as single-loop and double-loop learnings.

Argyris and Schön (1996) advanced the concepts of single-loop and double-loop learning that are relevant to knowledge generation for both individuals and organizations. Single-loop learnings are instrumental learnings that lead to improved performance without changing underlying values, norms, or strategies regarding current practices (Argyris & Schön, 1996). Double-loop learnings question underlying values, norms, or strategies, ultimately leading to changes in how and/or why certain practices are being done (Argyris & Schön, 1996).

Double loop-learning transpires when the inquiry results in changes to individual or organizational values of "theories-in-use" (Argyris & Schön, 1996). Theories-in-use are the patterns that are implicit in individual or organizational behaviors and can be compared to "espoused theory" (Argyris & Schön, 1996). Espoused theory represents the strategies and values that individuals or organizations communicate to explain their actions (Argyris & Schön, 1996). Fundamentally, espoused theory represents the notion of "what we say we do," which can be compared to theories-in-use that signifies "what we actually do" (Senge, 2006).

The notions of single-loop and double-loop learning complement networked improvement communities because PDSA cycles and other network activities could lead to either single-loop or double-loop learnings. Both types of learning would be beneficial. However, single-loop learning on its own may not be enough to meet the specific purposes of networked improvement communities. Networks are intended to solve complex problems of practice, which may require educators to change their underlying values, norms, and/or strategies regarding their current practices, thus, necessitating a need for double-loop learnings. Therefore, Argyris and Schön's (1996) organizational learning theory provides a useful model for conceptualizing learning.

The book's next six chapters provide a narrative of the network's first year and the subsequent learnings. The case study is a real-world account of the network's journey, including the challenges that arose and our attempts to deal with them. Chapters 3 and 4 are chronological and tell the story of the network. Chapters 5, 6, and 7 go more in-depth into notable findings. Last, Chapter 8 summarizes the findings and shares lessons learned. This case study serves as a practical example for those hoping to launch similar endeavors. Pseudonyms are used to protect the confidentiality of all individuals and schools.

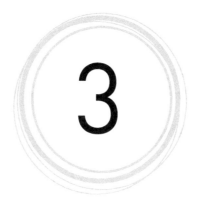

The Beginnings
of a Network

In September 2016, I was sitting in my advisor's office discussing potential dissertation topics, again. It had been months, and I still had not landed on the right one. As an applied researcher and program evaluator for the past 15 years of my career, I had little interest in the theoretical. Still struggling to find something practical, yet significant enough to warrant a dissertation, I was sure this meeting would end no closer to an answer.

But then my advisor told me the University had recently received a grant from a philanthropic foundation to establish a networked improvement community. The grant's purpose was to construct a network of schools that will work together in a sustained partnership for improvement in teaching and learning in diverse K–12 schooling contexts. A world-renowned public institution, the University had a strong commitment to social justice and improving the quality of the education workforce in today's urban schools. They had pledged to develop a math networked improvement community grounded in improvement science for its disciplined inquiry framework. I was intrigued. A newly forming network using improvement science theories in a practical application? We had found my topic.

This chapter, along with Chapter 4, describes the narrative of the network. In doing so, it provides details about how to initiate an improvement science network and build capacity, including how and why certain decisions were made.

In this chapter, I cover:

- Building the Network Hub Team
- Building the Rest of the Team

- Recruiting the Network Schools

- Launching the Network

- Our Own Challenge: Decision to Separate From the Larger Network

Building the Network Hub Team

Introducing Jackie

My advisor connected me with Jackie. She managed the grant and was charged with developing and running the network. We agreed that in addition to researching the network for my dissertation, I would also help her coordinate it as a graduate student researcher. Neither of us had experience building a networked improvement community.

Jackie was an associate dean in the University's Graduate School of Education. In that role, she oversaw programs that connected the University with local neighborhood and community schools and had substantial experience directing school initiatives and providing professional development. She started her career as a high school math teacher for 12 years. During her time as a teacher, she participated in the University Mathematics Project, which provided professional development for teachers. She was asked to serve as the director of the Mathematics Project and eventually transitioned into the full-time director of it. Jackie was also part of a team that launched a University Center focused on linking K–12 research and practice. She became its first executive director and then became the Associate Dean of the Graduate School of Education. Jackie's focus was always on supporting teachers and schools. As she tells it:

> So I was the Executive Director of the Center, which was about the intersection of research and practice. I was faculty in the teacher education program. I supported and prepared teachers going into the teaching of secondary mathematics. I did that until about 4 years ago, when I became Associate Dean [of the Graduate School of Education]. So all of my work has been about engaging in schools, and looking at practice, and trying to work on how we inform practice, how we transform practice and schools. So that's where my experience comes from in this area.

Jackie was motivated to start the Network by her desire to support University-partnered schools.

> One of the challenges we faced was that we don't want to see our work at each of these schools . . . they kind of become silo-ed. Like, "Here's what we do here, here's what we do there." Once I was brought into this position as associate dean, I could see that there was this great need for bringing our work together. There were ways that we could learn from each of the schools. The experiences were all so different, but it didn't mean that there weren't things we could learn from each other. I wanted to figure out ways to bridge, to link, to learn from.

It was at that time that I started learning about improvement networks from Louis Gomez. It was his work. He started doing professional development with one of the schools around improvement networks and improvement science. That then led us to this discussion about how do we engage our other schools that the graduate school is connected to. [It] made us start thinking about this notion of network and what it means. He and I collaborated on trying to envision what it might look like. So that's how it got started.

Introducing Me

As a program evaluator by experience and training, I was, and still am, particularly interested in how to drive change through evaluative methods. Before undertaking my PhD, I served as the Manager for Research and Evaluation at a mid-to-large-size northern California school district, as part of a 2-year fellowship. Through that experience, I learned firsthand just how difficult it is to change an entrenched system and realized that rather than prioritizing outside knowledge we needed to find new ways to combine it with the collective knowledge and experience of the educators within. From that experience, I came to believe that sustainable, systemic change would require practical means for evaluators, researchers, and practitioners to work closely together. I was excited that this new networked improvement community was going to embrace these ideas.

After my fellowship concluded, I remained at the school district and led a project that implemented improvement science with the goal of improving the academic perseverance of middle school students. The project included principals (instead of teachers) from six middle schools and select district leaders. While we were able to strengthen relationships, and create a new culture of openness among the participating district staff and principals, the project never gained traction, and the group disbanded after 3 years. I deemed the effort a failure because nothing actionable resulted from it. Because of this experience, I had mixed feelings about my role in the new University network. I was excited for the opportunity to work closely with schools and share my evaluation experience, but I was reluctant to step up and lead our network. I did not want to fail again.

Building the Rest of the Team

Unsure of how to start a networked improvement community, I dove into the research. There was very little available. I turned to *Learning to Improve* (Bryk et al., 2015) and an article titled *A Framework for the Initiation of Networked Improvement Communities* (Russell et al., 2017). Step one: Build a network initiation team.

The network initiation team needed to serve several purposes. Its role was to recruit members, secure needed resources, and provide expertise in subject and improvement knowledge (Bryk et al., 2015). It also functioned to identify the problem of practice, analyze the system that contributes to the problem, develop an aim statement, and draft an initial theory of practice improvement (Bryk et al., 2015).

Jackie and I struggled with selecting our initiation team members. Who had relevant, complementary expertise, and the time needed to participate? Concurrently, we had to consider how to develop the aim statement and the initial theory of practice improvement (also known as a *driver diagram*). We debated whether to first develop the aim and initial driver diagram with the initiation team or to include all the network members in that development. Bryk and colleagues (2015) deem this a crucial initiation question:

> Do we convene a small team to orchestrate the up-front work of refining the problem and framing a prototypical driver diagram and measures? Or do we first assemble the interested partners and have them identify a problem to pursue together? This strikes us as important tactical decision. (p. 160)

The importance of this tactical decision could not be overstated. We grappled with this question for weeks, carefully deliberating the pros and cons. I knew from my previous work that teachers would not fully own a change idea, or the improvement science process, if they were not engaged at the onset (Rohanna, 2017). From her substantial school experience, Jackie also understood the importance of doing things with teachers, not to them. However, we recognized that convening the schools and teachers without an initial problem focus and asking them to build a driver diagram from scratch could be endless. We worried that teachers would find it challenging and frustrating while they were being asked to learn improvement science and find consensus with others. There was no perfect answer.

Just as we were about to make our difficult decision, we punted. (We would revisit this question again later.) We were not the only University network starting in the fall. Like us, the other network was interested in math and brought expertise in networked improvement communities and improvement science through their stronger affiliation with the Carnegie Foundation for the Advancement of Teaching. It made sense to join their network. We would be a subnetwork within their larger network.

Jackie and I still needed to build our own hub team to support our subnetwork. A core principle in improvement science is the inclusion of members with subject knowledge and members with profound knowledge (knowledge of how to improve) (Langley et al., 2009). As the improvement science specialist, I filled the latter role. But we still needed a math expert to provide the subject knowledge in addition to the teachers. We found that expertise in Tom.

Introducing Tom

Tom's vision for quality math instruction would prove to be fundamental to our network's work. He lived and breathed mathematics instruction. His doctorate and master's degrees were in education, with an emphasis on teacher education in multicultural society and teaching mathematics, respectively. He majored in mathematics in his undergraduate studies. Tom was a math coach when he joined the network. He worked for the University's Math Project and had an extensive background in math professional development and instruction. As he shared:

> *I have been a math facilitator, math consultant, math coach. All things math related. I've also been a professional development provider. I've been at many schools providing training and Cognitively Guided Instruction. A lot of our work in the Math Project has revolved around that. But, because of my background in middle school and high school math, I've also done a lot of professional development specific to that grade span of middle school and high school. I've also done a lot of coaching, both in elementary and middle school and high school. And I think a lot of that has been connected to, like, my prior life, which all of it was math teaching. I taught middle school and high school. I taught general math, Algebra 1, geometry, and calculus.*

Tom's passion for mathematics and coaching motivated him to join our network.

> *I'd received an email from Jackie basically inquiring about whether we knew, my colleague and I who worked for the Math Project, whether we knew someone who might be interested in a middle school and high school coaching. But I think it was very specific to algebra at that time, as well as another condition, which was whether the person would happen to have enough background in College Preparatory Mathematics, CPM, that program. I was like, "Ooh, that's me!" What excited me about it was just the emphasis on working with specifically algebra teachers. So when I saw Jackie at a school where we were providing professional development, Jackie and I happened to be in the same space, and we got to talking, and that was what got me even more interested in participating.*

Introducing Samantha

We also needed someone on our team who had relationships with the network's teachers and principals. Samantha was that person. At the University, Samantha was the director of an education initiative with University neighboring schools, two of who were in our network, and she had previously worked at another one. She was currently working toward an Education Doctorate Degree and had a Master's in Education with a teaching degree. Samantha saw an opportunity to liaise between the schools and us. She proactively offered to help facilitate access, advocate on the network's behalf, and importantly, represent the schools' perspective as we developed materials and activities for meetings. Samantha's own words best describe her passion for supporting schools:

> *[In my University position,] I'm responsible for bridging enrichment, enrollment, and working closely with principals. We have eight schools, and I'm responsible for four of them. Before that, I was at one of the network schools*

for about 7 years. So officially my job title there was Director of Bridging and Enrichment, but I was basically responsible for whatever the school needed. And that could be like working with the principal, to help with professional development, working with families, working with students, or helping place University resources at the school. Whether that's like student teachers or grants, volunteers, departments, donors, getting donors to come, helping distribute scholarships, to supporting kids, K–12, and beyond.

As Samantha tells it, joining our team was a "happy accident." Rather than being an "accident" however, Samantha had the foresight and motivation to understand her crucial role in the network:

So I first became aware when we started talking, you know. Jackie was talking about that there was a grant that she needed my help, like, talking to some of my schools. And at the time, I just thought it was another resource we were bringing. So I didn't even have any concrete plans. And then, as part of my job is to be on board, be on deck, to make sure that resources are happening at the schools. You know, schools are really chaotic and busy places. Sometimes everybody has the best intentions, but sometimes things don't happen just because either volunteers or groups don't really understand how schools work. Or schools really want the resources, but they just don't have somebody to be there, like, navigating and making sure that the scheduling works. And so I just kind of jumped on board that way. Then my role grew into something different, which is cool. But that's just sort of the nature of my job, is to always sort of be there in the beginning; to help facilitate and really to make sure things don't fall through the cracks.

Recruiting the Network Schools

Five schools were recruited to participate in our nascent network. They all resided in a large, metropolitan, urban school district. Like many urban public school districts, it was experiencing years of declining enrollment, possibly attributed, in part, to the growth of independent charter schools (Rich, 2012). Between 2001 and 2017, district enrollment had declined by 15% (California Department of Education [CDE], 2017b). Declining enrollment was also due to the socioeconomic factors of increasing area costs of living, including housing, and the demographic trend of lower birth rates.

The district had overall lower-than-desired academic performance. Little more than half the students in the secondary grades (55%) met or exceeded achievement standards for the state standards in English Language Arts. Less than a third (28%) met or exceeded the standards in math (CDE, 2017a).

The five network schools varied in their achievement scores, but all were concerned with improvement, especially in their math achievement. The schools had preexisting partnerships with the University, under Jackie's purview. She had relationships with the principals and personally called each one to ask if they would be interested in participating. They all said, "Yes." They were especially interested in the prospect of receiving additional math classroom coaching as part of their participation.

We commenced the network by meeting with the principals and teachers. From previous experience working with schools and conducting professional development, our team knew it would be difficult for teachers to use the improvement science tools on their own. We also knew it was hard for educators to meet and prioritize a continuous improvement process unless it was part of a set schedule (Rohanna, 2017). Thus, the purpose of these meetings was to hear their expectations, concerns, and hopes; clarify our commitment expectations; establish a structure and schedule; assure facilitation support; and importantly, establish our expectation that the University team would meet with the teachers at their schools, in-between the network convenings. These in-between meetings were a condition of their participation in the network. Maintaining this commitment would later prove to be trying at times.

Network School Descriptions

In total, 24 math teachers across five schools participated in the network during its first year. Five principals were asked to actively participate, but not all did. One assistant principal also participated.

Roosevelt School

Roosevelt was a district pilot school that was launched in the 2009–2010 school year and enjoyed a close University partnership. Its enrollment had tripled since opening. The teachers and administrators considered their school "unique" and were proud of their accomplishments. A commitment to social justice and their active role in the community were part of Roosevelt's self-identity.

For the most part, the school's math performance was higher than the overall district's (CDE, 2017a). More than 40% of the sixth graders (44%) and seventh graders (45%) met or exceeded standards, which was higher than the district's (28% for both grades). However, eighth-grade figures were lower than the district's (22% compared to 28%). While Roosevelt was outperforming the district, on average, there was still significant room for improvement: Fewer than half the students were meeting or exceeding standards, and Algebra I grades data from the past few years showed that approximately half the students were receiving Ds or Fs.

Through several years of working with the University on other improvement initiatives, Roosevelt teachers already had exposure to and/or experience with improvement science tools and processes. Their principal valued and promoted a strong culture of improvement and expected the teachers to conduct PDSA cycles. However, some of the teachers expressed concerns that they still did not completely understand the process and suspected that they were possibly doing it incorrectly. This turned out to be an accurate self-assessment, based on my observation of one of their in-school meetings in October of that first year.

During this meeting, the math teachers, who spanned multiple grade levels, were sharing results from a PDSA cycle they had conducted independently from the network. They had one collective PDSA form for all the teachers. Issues became obvious when they tried to find consensus and/or identify strategies that were conducive to each teacher's specific needs. The teachers taught a variety of courses, and their one-size-fits-all PDSA form was not practical. Additionally, they were unclear what their prediction for the cycle was, or why there even was one. Thus, there was still substantial room to improve in their improvement science skills. Despite that, their existing knowledge assisted them greatly throughout the year, and they had in-school work structures already in place. Their foundation was more developed than other schools. It was something to build on.

Their network attendance was fairly consistent throughout the year. One teacher, who had been on leave missed most of the meetings in the fall but returned by January. Two other teachers missed a couple meetings each, but the rest of the group attended all the network meetings.

Marshall School

Marshall was a school that aimed to provide its students with quality instruction and "experiences in art, technology, leadership, and athletics." The school's enrollment declined substantially between 2005 and 2015 (66%) but was starting to grow again in recent years.

The school's math performance was a little higher than the overall district's (CDE, 2017a). A little more than a third of the sixth graders (34%) and seventh graders (38%) met or exceeded standards. Thirty-one percent of eighth graders met or exceeded standards. While Marshall was outperforming the district in those grade levels, there was clearly still cause for concern, since more than half the students were not meeting standards.

Marshall's team consisted of six teachers who attended network convenings consistently; however, we struggled to schedule time to work with them between those meetings. Even though we had emphasized this expectation to the administrator and the teachers at our first in-school meeting, we had difficulty getting them to follow through on that commitment. They could not confirm a consistent day and time for the intermediate meetings and often did not reply to Samantha's email. We were only able to work with the teachers at their school four times throughout the year, and that was due to Samantha's diligence, tenacity, and relationships with them.

The administrator attendance at meetings was inconsistent. He attended the first network convening and a portion of one other meeting in April. Importantly, at our first meeting with him and his teachers in October, he expressed concerns about following the improvement science process. He wanted flexibility to continue following his own approach for working with his teachers rather than strictly following the network's process. Through this conversation and others, I suspected that he did not value the improvement science process, which likely contributed to the lack of urgency in scheduling in-school meetings.

Middleview School

Middleview was a school going through a major transition. At one point in its history, it had been a prominent neighborhood school. The school experienced a sharp decline in enrollment during the 2000s with its enrollment falling by more than half (68%) between 2001 and 2011 (CDE, 2017b). After that, enrollment continued to slowly drop. The decline in enrollment was mostly due to the large number of charters opening in the surrounding neighborhood. By 2016, it was a school in crisis and entered a new partnership with the University with hopes of restoring its once-held position as a leading neighborhood school.

Middleview was described as a high needs school. According to those connected with the school and the CDE data (2017b), it had a relatively high population of students in foster care, students classified as special education and/or having disabilities, and English Language Learners. Less than 1% in any of the grades met or exceeded the math standards (CDE, 2017a). With the University as a partner, the school was in the process of rebuilding its instructional capacity. The year prior to the network year, the school only had two permanent math teachers—sixth and eighth grade. Seventh grade had a long-term substitute for the year. It was, by far, the most challenged school in the network.

When the network started, the school still did not have all its math teacher positions filled with permanent staff. Two teachers attended the first network meeting. Of those two, one was a first-year teacher. Another beginning teacher, who did not attend the first meeting, was also added to the team. A third teacher, also in their first year, joined the school in the winter. Because of this significant instructional transition, and their high needs population, Jackie suggested we take a different approach than the other schools. Our plan was to invite them into the network and support them, but we would allow them to take the lead rather than insist they follow the same structures as the other schools. We did not visit their principal, who was in his third year leading the school, to clarify commitment expectations before the network started. We assumed that full participation in this process would be too overwhelming for the teachers, so we did not dictate that they focus on the to-be-determined shared problem of practice, and we did not initially ask them to schedule regular school meetings with us.

Notably, the assumptions we made about Middleview turned out to be wrong and had unforeseen consequences. Our hands-off approach allowed the district's own continuous improvement initiative to swoop in. The teachers met regularly as part of their process, thus, making it more difficult for them to meet with us.

Middleview's principal did not attend any convenings even though he was regularly invited. Participation in the network by the teachers was inconsistent. Administration was concerned that leaving their classrooms for the full-day network meetings was too disruptive for their students. More than once, they only allowed one or two teachers to attend rather than the whole team. Most of the teachers missed many network meetings. We did not meet with them regularly at their schools, although we did attend other meetings at their school with them.

Sawyer School

After a steady decline in enrollment, Sawyer was a school on the rise (CDE, 2017b). For years, parents from the neighborhood chose other schools for their children. The current principal, who had been in the position for a few years, had been working to rebuild goodwill and trust with the surrounding community and staff, and now, the school was experiencing an increase in attendance from local families.

On average, the school's math performance was a little lower than the overall district's. About a third of the sixth graders (31%) met or exceeded standards, which was similar to the district's percentage (CDE, 2017a). However, its seventh- and eighth-grade student percentages were less than the district, with 18% and 11% meeting or exceeding standards (CDE, 2017a).

When the first network meeting convened, the math department was short in permanent math teachers. The principal was still in the process of "right-sizing" the staff—some existing teachers were let go, and new teachers were being brought onboard. The initial math team who attended the first network meeting consisted of two veteran teachers and one new teacher. During the year, two other teachers joined the team. One teacher was already at the school but was teaching both math and science courses, and a new teacher joined in late fall.

Attendance was inconsistent at the fall network convenings. While the whole team attended the first meeting, and included their assistant principal who oversaw math, only one teacher and the assistant principal attended the second meeting, and they had to leave early. No one attended the third meeting. The drop off in attendance at the second meeting could be attributed to it falling on the same day as their parent-teacher conferences. However, their complete absence at the third meeting was due to a lack of communication with the teachers. They were either unaware of, or had forgotten, about the meeting. The assistant principal expressed his apologies.

However, attendance improved and was consistent during the second part of the year, after they had expanded their team. Most of the teachers came to the meetings. One did not attend in the winter and spring because she was participating in a teacher fellowship program that required her to miss more full days.

Central School

Central could be described as stable and "welcoming." Its principal had been there for years. Both the teachers and the principal depicted a diverse staff that reflected the student body. Their population of students included those from the surrounding neighborhood, as well as other areas.

Following the district trend, Central was experiencing declining enrollment (CDE, 2017b); however, during my time working with the school, I never heard anyone express concern, unlike at the other two schools. This is likely because the decline occurred to a smaller and slower degree than the others, and it still retained a healthy size (1,564 students).

According to the eleventh-grade math state assessment data, Central performed higher than the district in math (35% versus 24% meeting or exceeding standards) (CDE, 2017a). Yet for obvious reasons, there were still concerns: Only about a third of the students were at or above standards. Additionally, almost half the students were failing ninth-grade algebra.

There was a "nice" mix of older and newer teachers in the school. Its three ninth-grade algebra teachers who participated in the network represented that nice mix. One of the teachers was newer, having been there for 3 years, while the other two were veteran teachers. While all three teachers initially attended the network convening meetings, one of the veteran teachers attended sparsely in the spring. For the most part, his lack of attendance was not explained. While he was out of town for one meeting, he was expected at the other three meetings by his principal yet did not show up.

At Central, the principal was very involved and supportive of the network. He rarely missed a meeting. He provided time during the school day for the three teachers to meet with us regularly during a conference period. He alternated that time so the teachers, who did not all have one common conference period, would take turns missing class. He sought coverage for the teachers during those meetings, which for the most part, occurred every 2 weeks. Before those school meetings, our University team would also meet with him to get his perspective on what we were going to cover in the meeting (and sometimes the upcoming network convening). He helped us better understand his teachers' needs and their concerns about the network process.

Launching the Network

As previously described, we were a subnetwork within a larger network when we first launched. Jackie and I made the decision to be part of the larger network because of their expertise in starting networked improvement communities and strong connections to the Carnegie Foundation for the Advancement of Teaching. We had none of those advantages.

The large network was comprised of 16 schools, excluding ours. They were all high schools, while our schools and teachers represented sixth through ninth grades. Their network focused solely on high school algebra. Like them, we had originally planned to focus on algebra, but during early conversations with our schools they pointed out how crucial it was to involve the other grades when considering problems around algebra. They were highlighting a systems problem. Jackie explained:

And they pushed that Algebra I is also in middle school. The issues surrounding it don't start in eighth grade or ninth grade or with Algebra I. It's everything that happens before, you know. So that was the thinking that, while at first we thought it was going to be all about Algebra I, we were pushed by the schools. Algebra I is an issue, but it's also what happens in the previous level.

Because we subsumed into the larger network, our network adhered to their training activities. Their team took the lead on organizing and planning the monthly network meetings. We provided input and communicated with our five schools, but did not play a role in deciding what content would be delivered at the network meetings.

We did, however, have a blueprint for building the improvement science capacity of our five school teams. Per my initial research, we knew it was crucial to determine the objective(s) at the outset when building evaluation capacity (Preskill & Boyle, 2008). As described earlier in Chapter 1, improvement science is a form of participatory evaluation (Christie et al., 2017; Cousins & Earl, 1992). As such, there were three broad capacity building objectives to consider: knowledge and understanding, skills and behaviors, and affective or attitudes (Labin et al., 2012; Preskill & Boyle, 2008). Our primary objective in the first year was for teachers to learn processes and embed them in their schools. Thus, our focus was on building skills and behaviors and transferring those skills to their work context. While gaining knowledge and understanding seems like a notable first step, we took the position that our team's improvement science specialist (me) would provide that expertise by facilitating the improvement science work at the schools. Of course, we were also concerned with attitudes. We knew behaviors would be more likely to stick if teachers saw the value in this work. Fortunately, as we found out later, Tom's math expertise provided this aspect.

Understanding the Problem

As discussed in Chapter 1, the first phase in improvement science is identifying and understanding a problem of practice before developing solutions for improving it. The larger network's teams planned and led activities at the monthly convenings to this end.

Network Convenings, August to November

The network began with a convening of all the principals. This occurred in August after school started. Three fall network convenings followed. The purpose of these meetings was to teach the schools improvement tools and methods to define a common problem of practice, establish an aim statement, and eventually, develop a driver diagram. Tables 3.1 through 3.3 outline the content taught and the activities facilitated at each of these meetings.

TABLE 3.1 ● September Network Convening Content and Activities

Network groupings	September meeting sessions/content	Activities
8 a.m. to 12 p.m. (All network schools)	Introduction of network	Presentation of concepts
	6 Core Principles of Improvement	Presentation of concepts
	Identifying the problem	Presentation of concepts; Brainstorming landmark problems by school; Fishbone Diagram; 5 Whys
	Empathy interviews	Presentation of concepts; active listening exercise; practice empathy interviews
12 p.m. to 3 p.m. (Only our 5 schools)	Real-world example of school improvement process	Presentation by a principle
	Reflection on plans for own improvement	Discussions within school teams
	Understanding the problem	Using one tool (Fishbone Diagram, or 5 Whys) continued brainstorming around their landmark problem in school teams
	Reflection	Whole group reflection

Before the October convening, the large network (including our schools) were given several pieces of homework to complete:

- Continue working on their fishbone diagram, and possibly include other colleagues.

- Gather any data related to their landmark problem and bring to the next meeting.

- Conduct empathy interviews and/or observations with at least two people in their school.

- Find and read literature associated with their landmark problem to gain an understanding of what the field says regarding this problem.

We met with all our schools, except Middleview, between the October and November convenings. The primary purpose of these meetings was to outline our expectations, learn about their expectations, and facilitate the fishbone diagram, also known as a *Cause and Effect diagram*, as a part of their root cause analysis. The fishbone diagram is a visual tool for causal analysis, whereby the facilitator asks participants to brainstorm potential causes of a problem and group them together to identify themes. To facilitate these meetings, I developed kits that included Post-It notes, a hand-made 14 x 18.5 inch fishbone diagram, and fishbone diagram examples. The secondary purpose was to establish network-related work structures within the school.

We knew time was a scarce commodity for teachers. Even with the best intentions, it is difficult for educators to find the time and energy to commit to an improvement endeavor. As enticement, we offered to help them complete their homework and prepare for the meetings, if they agreed to commit to one or two set meetings a month. This tactic created a set time for network-related work and minimized any additional work for them outside of that set time.

The schools were not given any homework between the October and November meetings. We continued to meet with our schools individually.

TABLE 3.2 ● October Network Convening Content and Activities

October meeting (8 a.m.–2 p.m.) sessions/content	Activities
Fishbone and high-leverage problems	Presentation of concepts and examples; re-working fishbone diagrams in school teams; paired schools shared with each other; whole group share-out, one school at a time
Finding a shared network problem of practice	Identify, categorize, and prioritize potential problems of practice through school discussions and whole group voting
Further prioritize top problems	Effort and benefit continuum prioritization, within school teams and then as a network
Fishbone on one of the two top priorities (lack of prerequisite skills and mindsets)	Redo fishbone in school teams; shared in small inter-school groups
Pareto chart	Presentation of concept and directions

TABLE 3.3 ● November Network Convening Content and Activities

November meeting (8 a.m.–3 p.m.) sessions/content	Activities
Reminder of the network process and purpose	Presentation
Continue causal analysis with fishbone diagrams	School teams revisited fishbone diagrams from the last network meeting
Pareto charts	Presentation of concepts

Process maps	Presentation of concepts; scaffolded exercise; school teams developed their own
Aim statements	Presentation of concepts; school teams developed their own

Our Own Challenge: Decision to Separate From the Larger Network

From the beginning, we were able to structure our sub-network differently from the larger network. Our subnetwork was small and manageable. We had five schools and existing relationships with them. With our core team—an improvement science specialist, a math coach, and a liaison with knowledge of and relationships with the schools—we had the resources to support our schools in both the improvement science and math content.

The larger network also had a team but was limited by resources. They supported 16 schools, but only had two or three people available for additional support within those schools. Unlike our team, no one in their network had math instruction content expertise, and only one, other than the project director, had improvement science experience. During our meetings together, they acknowledged this made it challenging to provide the additional within-school support that our network provided. However, they did make themselves available for individual school support. Initially, it was by request, and then eventually, they began making more regular visits.

Due to our size and the support of our team, our network progressed more quickly than the larger network. As previously discussed, we met with the schools individually between large network meetings to facilitate the improvement science activities. We also engaged them in collaborative dialogue around math instructional issues. By the end of the second meeting (October), it was clear our schools were further along because we had already facilitated some of the activities that were occurring at the network meetings. So much so that some of the activities at the second meeting felt redundant to our teachers. At the third meeting in November, one of our principals questioned the purpose of doing a fishbone diagram again because, through our in-school support, they had already progressed past the causal analysis and were beginning to brainstorm potential drivers on how to improve Algebra I pass rates. It had become apparent we would have to reevaluate our participation in the larger network. This reconsideration was based on a few factors:

- Our teachers were frustrated. By November, they had spent 3 months trying to understand the problem of practice. Although we did not want to rush to find solutions, we risked losing their interest and motivation if they did not get to try something new in their classroom soon.

- We had concerns about the direction of the larger network's common problems of practice. Both problems were centered on student deficits: students' gaps in knowledge and lack of growth mindsets (students and teachers). We felt the teachers needed more direction framing a problem of practice that was within their locus of control and integrated with their instructional practices.

- The schools were not uniting around a common problem of practice. At the end of the third network meeting, the schools developed aim statements (i.e., measurable goals for improvement). Three of our five schools shared their aims. One school's team did not write one because of internal disagreements. The fifth school did not attend the meeting. The foci of the three aim statements were disparate and distant: improving student problem-solving skills, improving the percentage of students passing Algebra I, and improving the process of student grouping in the CPM curriculum. Our schools were not moving closer in their focus. They were actually moving further apart.

Given those developments, we realized we needed to bring more cohesion and a common purpose within our five schools. So we made the decision to separate from the larger network and relaunch our small network.

Conclusion

Launching a network requires a hub team with multiple perspectives and areas of expertise, as well as an understanding of the various contexts and challenges faced by the participants. Ideally, those who support networks can meet individually with schools to learn about their own unique challenges and desires in addition to meeting with the network as a whole. Meeting more frequently and facilitating improvement activities can also help the process move more quickly, and thus hopefully assuage frustration that is likely to arise from an intentionally thoughtful process that takes time.

Questions for Discussion

1. Why is important to understand context (e.g., who is on the team, the individual schools) when leading change?

2. If you were leading this network, who would you have included on the hub team? Whose perspective might be missing?

3. What are you own experiences, either leading or participating, in a change initiative where there was a tension between following a deliberate process and the desire to take action?

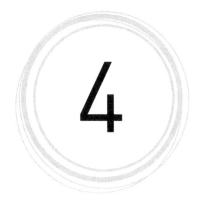

The Re-Launch

At this moment, I valued Tom and Samantha's expertise even more as we prepared to separate from the larger network. I was also more confident in my improvement science expertise. While participating in those larger network meetings, I realized my knowledge was on par with theirs. I even wondered if I had a distinct advantage in my program evaluation background. My comfort and deep understanding around disciplined inquiry, theories of change, and data and measures, along with my experience working for a school district, would inform my efforts to unpack technical ideas, and hopefully, render them more accessible for teachers.

Even with an amazing team and a newfound confidence in my improvement science knowledge, I was still unsettled about next steps. It was December. To keep momentum, we needed our teachers experimenting in their classroom by early February, which left us with one network meeting in January. *How were we going to develop a new shared problem of practice, a common aim, and a driver diagram and change ideas to test in less than 2 months?*

In this chapter, I cover:

- Seeking the Counsel of Others

- Developing the Network's Theory of Improvement

- Taking Action Through PDSAs

- The Network's Outcome, End of Year 1

Seeking the Counsel of Others

I sought the counsel of another established math networked improvement community and arranged a conference call with the two people who led that network. They shared their experiences and provided valuable guidance.

Having previous experience introducing improvement science to principals, I was unsurprised by two experiences that they shared because they mirrored my own. First, they purposely minimized the importance of the driver diagram. Teachers were not engaged by it and became bored. They suggested that I move the driver diagram to the background rather than the foreground of the work. Second, they were flexible with the requirement that Plan, Do, Study, Act (PDSA) cycles be short iterative cycles. They were comfortable with the longer cycles (i.e., more than a couple weeks), which seemed to embrace the idea of creating a longer plan rather than testing small changes. Ironically, these were my two non-negotiables.

I understood their sentiment toward driver diagrams. It reminded me of my previous experience working with middle school principals trying to improve the academic perseverance of students. The principals' eyes would glaze over any time I presented the driver diagram. It seemed too technical to them. As a result, I, too, minimized its importance. The principals all had access to it, but I rarely showed it after its initial introduction. The result: They never remembered our theory for improvement and did not develop change ideas intentionally aligned with it, if at all. Thus, it was not serving its theory of change purpose.

Also based on previous experience, I was resolved to short iterative PDSA cycles. The intention behind PDSA cycles is learning, generated from the cycles (Langley et al., 2009). Each time a small change is tested, a new learning is generated. Thus, the formal cycle of learning is the same length as the PDSA cycle. With my former academic perseverance project, the learning was slow. The principals committed to one PDSA cycle in the fall and one in the spring. They met after each cycle, shared the results, and reflected together. Beneficial, yes, but not likely to be truly transformative. Rather than generating rapid incremental learnings, completing cycles that fit within their schedule became the goal. During that project, we lost sight of the PDSA purpose when we tried to adapt it to the school setting. I did not want to make the same mistake twice.

I also subscribed to a view from the Toyota Kata (Rother, 2010). We were in this for the long haul. Changing organizational learning behaviors meant building skills and establishing structures, routines, and habits (Preskill & Boyle, 2008; Rother, 2010). And it was important to teach the *right* habits (Rother, 2010). Being too accommodating could lead to the wrong habits. Through my experience with Roosevelt, I realized that the wrong habits could lead to extreme frustration if teachers were authentically engaging in the improvement science process, but then getting stuck, or not seeing promised results. Of course, the trick is understanding when to be flexible and when to be strict, when to adhere to the rigorousness of the process and when to make adaptations. For me, I drew that line at this whole network's purpose: generating meaningful learnings that could solve complex problems of practice. I wanted to accelerate learning.

I shared my perspective and my own commitment to keeping the rigor of these two improvement science processes with the two people who led the other network. They offered two invaluable pieces of advice:

1. Own the driver diagram. This meant letting the hub develop it rather than trying to bring the teachers to consensus.

2. Establish a math instructional vision. This meant giving the math expert (Tom) a larger role in the network convenings so that he could more explicitly guide teachers' experimentation in their classrooms.

Developing the Network's Theory of Improvement

Tom, Samantha, and I brought these two pieces of advice together as we developed the essential network elements needed to propel our small network forward. Once again, we faced the initiation team question that Jackie and I had dodged (or so we thought). The tactical question that Bryk and his colleagues (2015) consider essential:

Do we convene a small team to orchestrate the up-front work of refining the problem and framing a prototypical driver diagram and measures? Or do we first assemble the interested partners and have them identify a problem a problem to pursue together? (p. 160)

Even though only a few months had passed, we were in a better position to answer this question. Our answer: Do a hybrid. Because we facilitated activities and conversations at our schools—we had artifacts from their causal analysis and had even begun drafting drivers with some of the schools—we knew what problems they had identified and some of the instructional issues they struggled with. We gathered their fishbone diagrams, process maps, beginning driver diagrams, and our notes. We three would use these artifacts to refine the problem and develop the preliminary driver diagram. We felt this hybrid strategy was advantageous because it represented our teachers' views and experiences, without placing the burden on them to learn and develop a driver diagram, or to find consensus, both within their own teams, and among the other schools. We would serve as the consensus-makers. Yet we were still uncertain how they would receive it. *Would they embrace it as their own?*

Before establishing the driver diagram, we needed to determine the network problem of practice. We had two criteria: teacher-focused rather than student deficit-focused and sufficient flexibility for each school's needs, while begetting coherence among them.

I remembered something one of our former large network colleagues said at a planning meeting. Several of us were sharing our concerns with the two initial problems of practice selected by the large network. He articulated that the real issue was the "lack of alignment between the learning needs of kids and teacher skills." He was right. In one form or another, our teachers had expressed that they were unsure how to deal with incoming students who did not have prerequisite math knowledge, lacked problem-solving skills, struggled to make mathematical connections with real-world applications, and/or simply had no interest in mathematics. We also heard many of them express that today's students processed information differently because of the Internet and social media.

This provided an opportunity to pivot from what teachers perceived students were lacking to the real issue: Our current instructional practices were not aligned with students' learning needs today. While possibly too broad of a problem statement for improvement science purists, it provided coherence with flexibility, and importantly, a path forward for our teachers from diverse schools who represented multiple grade levels.

Initial Network Problem of Practice: Our current practices are not aligned with students' learning needs today. Many students are failing math.

It was almost poetic that shortly after New Year's Day, Tom, Samantha, and I "locked ourselves in a room" to develop the brand new initial driver diagram. We first agreed on a potential network aim. Rather than set measurable targets for the schools, we decided on a global aim that was broad. We would let the schools set their own targets, again recognizing that each school had different needs.

Initial Network Global Aim Statement: Our practices actively engage students in math and meet their variety of learning needs. We know we're improving when more students are learning and passing math classes with a C grade or better.

Tom's notions of math instruction guided our development of the driver diagram. During the fall, Tom sent me a copy of the National Council of Teachers of Mathematics (2014) report, *Principles to Actions: Ensuring Mathematical Success for All.* We made connections between specific passages and what we were hearing at the schools. Importantly, the report also depicted an image of effective teaching and learning in mathematics.

An excellent mathematics program requires effective teaching that engages students in meaningful learning through individual and collaborative experiences that promote their ability to make sense of mathematical ideas and reason mathematically. (p. 7)

With this report and the school artifacts, Tom, Samantha, and I drafted a preliminary driver diagram. We sequestered ourselves in one of the University's classrooms, equipped with the ubiquitous wall-sized whiteboard at the front of the room. They sat at the student tables, while I stood in front. I facilitated the discussion—asking Tom and Samantha questions, pushing their thinking, and pressing them to explain why one action would lead to another—while I jotted down ideas on the whiteboard and sketched out how they were linked, working and reworking primary and secondary driver descriptions. I hoped that we would complete the diagram, but at the end of the third hour, in what was supposed to be a 2-hour meeting, we had only drafted one primary and several secondary drivers. And as Samantha stated, "My head hurts." Her comment reminded me of the time I taught a friend how to create a logic model. After 2 hours, he said that he could not think anymore. I shared that story with Samantha and offered that maybe I took the effort for granted. My brain had been trained to think in terms of causal pathways from years of evaluating programs. She likened creating the driver diagram to training for a marathon: You have to start small. You cannot just go out and run 26 miles. You run a couple miles and build up endurance. For you (me), it is like you can already run the marathon. I reflected on her comment. Theories of change and driver diagrams are technical and complex. *Why would we ever expect educators to be capable of doing this with no experience and little training?*

It took a second rigorous 3-hour meeting to complete the driver diagram. Armed with the phrase "possibly wrong and definitely incomplete" (Bryk et al., 2015), we felt that we had a solid preliminary driver diagram that could be shared with the network. Our roll-out plan was to detail how we created the diagram from their perspectives and artifacts and then solicit their feedback for revisions. Figure 4.1 shows the initial driver diagram.

Even though we were satisfied with the preliminary driver diagram, I was still left with one nagging feeling. It was not very systems-oriented in the traditional sense of improvement science.

One of the four tenets of profound knowledge is the knowledge of systems (Christie et al., 2017; Langley et al., 2009). As mentioned previously, profound knowledge is defined "as the interplay of theories of systems, variation, knowledge, and psychology" (Deming, cited in Langley et al., 2009, p. 75). Systems knowledge refers to the interdependence of departments, people, and processes within an organization. Langley and colleagues (2009) assert that "understanding the organization as a system" is one of the components of a system of improvement (p. 312).

The idea of systems thinking in education was a concept I grappled with frequently. The term itself, *systems*, was very abstract to me, even though I understood its significance. For example, a school district's assessment policy could inadvertently reduce the number of instructional hours in a classroom, or that the incoming mathematical knowledge of new seventh-grade students greatly depends on the sixth-grade math instruction. Yet in education, these interdependent policies, people, and processes are often outside the teacher's locus of control. For me, the system needed to be bounded by the people in our room, who were primarily teachers.[1]

---

[1]As discussed in Chapter 2 and Chapter 8, I have since evolved in my thinking around systems and systems thinking and now understand the importance of both bounding the system while also addressing the unique dynamics of complex systems and potential patterns that hinder change.

FIGURE 4.1 ● Network Driver Diagram in Year 1

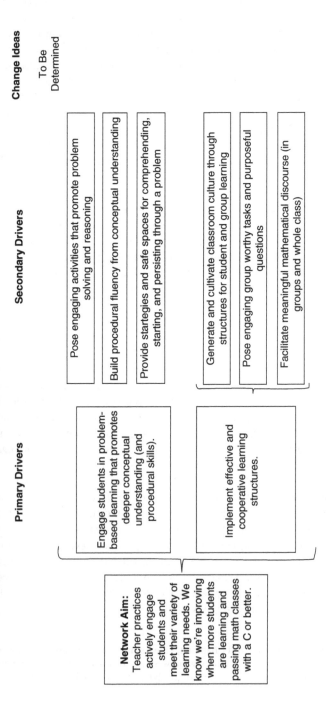

Primary Drivers

Secondary Drivers

Change Ideas

To Be
Determined

Network Aim:
Teacher practices
actively engage
students and
meet their variety of
learning needs. We
know we're improving
when more students
are learning and
passing math classes
with a C or better.

Engage students in problem-
based learning that promotes
deeper conceptual
understanding (and
procedural skills).

Implement effective and
cooperative learning
structures.

Pose engaging activities that promote problem
solving and reasoning

Build procedural fluency from conceptual understanding

Provide startegies and safe spaces for comprehending,
starting, and persisting through a problem

Generate and cultivate classroom culture through
structures for student and group learning

Pose engaging group worthy tasks and purposeful
questions

Facilitate meaningful mathematical discourse (in
groups and whole class)

Langley and colleagues (2009) assert this idea that systems need to have boundaries: "The larger the system, the more difficult it is to optimize" (p.78). This phrase reminded me of an observation shared by one the principals from my previous project. During one of those meetings, I projected a slide with the Central Law of Improvement: "Every system is perfectly designed to deliver the results it produces" and explained the importance of interdependent parts of a whole (Langley et al., 2009, p. 79). One principal immediately spoke up and lamented: Every time someone brings up systems, they never mention that there are a lot of parts outside of their control. For example, family life is part of this system, but they cannot control that. His obvious frustration and disdain toward systems thinking had stuck with me, years later.

Remembering that previous experience, I felt the system needed to be small and manageable. Because our network was very instructionally focused, we considered teachers' classrooms to be their systems. I also resolved to drop the abstract term *systems* when talking with educators and instead replace it with a more concrete depiction (i.e., the classroom). While this all made sense from a practical standpoint, it was still unsettling. I worried that the boundary was too small from a more traditional systems thinking sense. After returning to that idea of where to draw the line between rigor and flexibility, I chose flexibility. Narrowing the system was more likely to propel us forward and foster learnings rather than inhibit us.

Taking Action Through PDSAs

As we relaunched, Tom, Samantha, and I organized to support teachers with developing new strategies and implementing PDSAs. We held four network convenings between January and May. For each of those meetings, we established objectives and planned relevant activities and content, shown in Tables 4.1 through 4.4. We posted meeting materials on our newly developed network website. We continued to meet with schools between the convenings as we did during the first half of the year.

Network Convenings, January to May

January Convening

Our goal was to have the schools identify a change idea aligned with the driver diagram that they could experiment with for their first PDSA cycle. We wanted them to start and complete the cycle within 2 weeks of that first meeting. Toward that meeting goal, we provided the following content and professional development.

Because we were still concerned with whether our teachers would accept the problem of practice, aim statement, and the driver diagram as their own, we explicitly described how we developed these network essentials from their artifacts and dialogue. To our surprise and gratification, we received positive

TABLE 4.1   ●   January Network Convening Content and Activities

January meeting (8 a.m.–3 p.m.) sessions/content	Activities
Introduction. Overview of the network's purpose	Presentation of our progress thus far, and a timeline
Network problem of practice and aim statement	Presentation of how we developed from their artifacts and discussions
Math professional development	Presentation and interactive activities where teachers experienced being the students for number sense routines
Driver diagram: What it is and how to use one	Presentation of concepts; school teams provided input on poster-sized diagram and selected drivers where they could improve
PDSA: What, why, and how	Presentation of concepts
Change idea	Introduction and brainstorming ideas in school teams.
Planning our PDSA cycles	Individual work time for teachers to plan PDSA cycle; fishbowl activity where two teachers shared and other teachers asked questions
Closing and reflection	Group reflection on the day

feedback regarding the driver diagram. Rather than dismissing it, the teachers expressed their appreciation that they were not forced to spend hours trying to create one and find consensus.

The teachers were asked to complete one PDSA cycle before the next network convening. Because we considered the classroom to be each teacher's system, each one was expected to complete and document their own PDSA cycle. That is, each teacher was asked to experiment with a new practice in their classroom, collect data that could inform whether they met their prediction regarding what they expected the new practice to achieve, reflect on those data, and then decide next steps.

We scheduled time to visit each school, except Middleview, who only had one teacher attend the January convening. The purpose of those meetings was for teachers to share the results of their PDSA cycles with each other and engage in inquiry and dialogue.

March Convening

When we visited the schools, I noticed that teachers were reluctant to ask each other questions. They seemed comfortable sharing their results, but often when I would ask, "What questions do you have for [teacher's name]," an awkward silence would fall over the room. In some cases, teachers would ask for some small clarification on what the other teacher had done or offer a suggestion for doing something differently next time, but I judged the conversations to be polite and benign. On a rare occasion, a teacher would really push another teacher's thinking, or forced them to justify why they had done something. This concerned me because the purpose of the PDSA cycle is to build knowledge through the reflection component, but the teachers seemed hesitant to dialogue with each other.

I worried that meaningful learnings would not occur if teachers were reluctant to ask deeper probing questions. The goal was not just individual learning but team learning that would then ascend to network learning (Engelbart, 1992). To build team learnings, individuals need reflection, inquiry, dialogue, and discussion skills (Senge, 2006). In my experience with cycles of inquiry in education, I have witnessed on numerous occasions (and participated in organizing) educators being brought together with expectations of engaging in inquiry and dialogue around some important issue and/ or data, yet no one had first taught them how to do it. *Why did we expect productive inquiry and dialogue to occur just because we put them all in a room together?* I reflected on this question and decided to explicitly teach them inquiry and dialogue skills.

Toward this end, the primary objective introduced at the March convening was instruction on how to engage in productive inquiry and dialogue, use those new skills to engage with teachers from other schools, and then plan their next PDSA cycles. Our secondary objective was to introduce data and practical measures, including classroom observation rubrics aligned to our driver diagram (developed by the hub team). For the productive inquiry and dialogue objective, we began by unpacking:

- what it means to engage in inquiry: asking questions, clarifying information, probing;

- what it means to engage in dialogue: exploration of issues through multiple people and/or perspectives, with a purpose of expanding our own individual understanding (Senge, 2006); and

- what it means to engage in productive inquiry and dialogue: improve their own practices and reflect on personal assumptions, potentially leading to a change in how they view and do things.

Next, we reviewed norms for engaging in productive inquiry and dialogue. We relayed our expectation that productive inquiry and dialogue is a skill that can be honed through practice. Our team modeled asking questions and gave teachers a chance to practice. We also provided a protocol to guide their inquiry and dialogue around PDSA cycles.

While we wanted teachers to engage in inquiry and dialogue with teachers from their own schools, it was also important for us to build this routine at the

TABLE 4.2 ● March Network Convening Content and Activities	
March meeting (8 a.m.–3 p.m.) sessions/content	Activities
Introduction. Reminder of network process, problem of practice, and aim statement	Presentation
Math professional development regarding implementing tasks that promote reasoning and problem solving and mathematical discourse (building on January's content)	Presentation and interactive activities where teachers experienced being the students for number sense routines
Engaging in productive inquiry and dialogue	Presentation of concepts; modeling and practicing inquiry and dialogue
PDSAs: Productive inquiry and dialogue across schools	Each teacher shared their PDSAs results with teachers from other schools; engaged in inquiry and dialogue using a protocol
Math professional development regarding making sense of students' thinking	Presentation and interactive activities
Planning next PDSA cycle	Individual work time for teachers to plan PDSA cycle
Data for improvement (practical measures) and system of measures	Presentation of concepts; brainstorming measures aligned to drivers; discussion around potential rubrics and run chart
Closing and reflection	Group reflection on the day

network level. To learn from other schools and build a network identity, teachers needed the opportunity to interact with one other. Therefore, teachers from different schools were strategically grouped together to engage in inquiry and dialogue. We grouped teachers who we felt would connect and build relationships, provide valuable guidance, and/or push each other's thinking.

Regarding the data and practical measures objective, teachers were asked to choose and test one classroom observation rubric and incorporate it into their current PDSA cycle. We sought to collect data regarding:

- engaging all students in mathematical activity,
- providing students with opportunities to explain their thinking, and
- providing opportunities for student-to-student questioning.

We assigned them the task of collecting data before, during, and after they tested their change idea, using a run chart format (similar to a line chart), which we developed as an Excel template for each of the rubrics. We hoped they would see variations between the day(s) when they implemented their change idea—an increase in student participation or mathematical discourse would be typically expected—compared to the other days. We also asked them to provide feedback on the rubric itself (e.g., whether it was suited for the task, whether the wording could be clarified or improved), along with other impressions. *Not one teacher* from any of our five schools did it. (Although two teachers did provide rubric feedback.)

I became aware of the situation before the April convening, thanks to our intervening in-school visits. During one of those visits, I asked if anyone had a chance to pilot the rubric or the run chart. Two teachers replied, "What is that?" Other teachers vaguely remembered the rubric exercise, but only after I described the procedure again to jog their memories. One teacher did remember the assignment and kept proclaiming, "It was the yellow piece of paper!" to the others, as if that were a better clue than my description. To her credit, some teachers did remember a yellow piece of paper. Unfortunately, no one could explain what was written on it.

To their defense, the rubric and run chart assignment was fairly technical. Some teachers stated they did not fully understand the directions. This confirmed what I observed at another school, a few days after the March convening. Two teachers were collecting data for the run chart, but on review, I realized they were not looking at the rubric descriptors while giving the ratings. Thus, they were not doing the activity as intended and also did not complete it.

Teachers also described feeling stressed. "It was a long day," they explained, during a time of year that already demanded a hectic pace at their schools due to the state testing calendar. As one teacher described:

> *I'm involved at the meetings [but] the minute I leave . . . I got to come [to school] and deal with who didn't learn what, and I got to re-teach . . . and [then] get ready for progress reports. All that.*

This was a common concern among teachers from all our schools. They described feeling "overwhelmed" and expressed concerns about missing a classroom day for a network convening, with state testing right around the corner. Even the "yellow paper" teacher revealed that she had forgotten the details of the assignment by the time she returned to her school. (One positive result of this meeting was the realization that teachers were more comfortable being candid and asking questions about technical content in this setting rather than in the network meetings.)

April Convening

We responded to their concerns. At the University team pre-meeting, we discussed a need to ease off the technical rigidity for the April convening. We designed activities where teachers would lead discussions, instead of being presented with technical ideas from us. Our recalibrated objectives for the upcoming convening would be: build relationships among schools, have teachers reflect on their own beliefs regarding student engagement in mathematics, and plan their last PDSA cycle of the school year.

We also continued to build network routines. Again, we grouped teachers from multiple schools and asked them to engage in inquiry and dialogue about their PDSA cycles using the established protocol. Additionally, at the end of this session, we asked the teachers to volunteer an inspiring practice that they heard in their group. The purpose of this activity was to highlight the learning that was occurring across schools and acknowledge the positive practices of our teachers.

TABLE 4.3 ● April Network Convening Content and Activities	
April meeting (8 a.m.–3 p.m.) sessions/content	**Activities**
Introduction. Reminder of network process, problem of practice, and aim statement	Presentation
Math professional development regarding implementing tasks that promote reasoning and problem solving and mathematical discourse	Presentation and interactive activities where teachers experienced being the students for number sense routines
Circles of engagement: Beliefs and assumptions around student engagement in the math classroom	Reading with protocol and facilitated small group discussion (mixed schools)
PDSAs: Productive inquiry and dialogue across schools	Time to complete their reflection from the last cycle; then each teacher shared their PDSAs results with teachers from other schools; engaged in inquiry and dialogue using a protocol
Spotlight from PDSA cycles	Whole group sharing out of inspiring practices heard from the PDSA discussion
Mapping change ideas to driver diagrams	Team activities to develop latest change idea, map it to the driver diagram, and present to whole group
Planning next PDSA cycle	Individual work time for teachers to plan PDSA cycle
Closing and reflection	Group reflection on the day

May Convening

Due to state testing occurring between the April and May convening, we were only able to meet with one school before the May convening. Our team also internally relaxed our requirement to complete the last PDSA cycle. Not only did we want to remove further pressure on the teachers, but I did not want them to be inauthentic to the process. By reviewing the shared PDSA forms on our network website and through discussions with several teachers, I knew many of them did not complete their last PDSA cycle. My fear was that they would say they conducted a PDSA cycle, without actually having completed one. Again, I had experienced this with the principals on my previous project. Therefore, even though we had asked them to plan a PDSA cycle at the April convening, we did not plan for them to share the results at the May convening. Our objectives for that final meeting were to continue developing a shared understanding of the network's purpose and to plan for next school year by setting measurable aims and revisiting our root cause analysis and driver diagram. Importantly, we also conducted a PDSA showcase—a recommendation from one of our teachers—that asked several teachers to demonstrate one of their change ideas from the year and/or a PDSA-related resource. The goal was for teachers to learn new ideas and/or strategies from each other, particularly

TABLE 4.4 ● May Network Convening Content and Activities

May meeting (8 a.m.–3 p.m.) sessions/content	Activities
Introduction. Reminder of network process and purpose	Presentation with reflection activity
Reflection on math professional development, and the idea of eliciting student thinking to respond to student needs	Presentation connecting all the math professional development from the previous meetings
Setting aim statement targets for upcoming year	School teams reviewed grades data for the previous 3 years and discussed
PDSA showcase	Teachers presented their change ideas and resources at stations, while other teachers rotated
Revisiting 5 Whys: Deepening our understanding of the problem	Facilitated 5 Whys activity with each school team
Revisiting driver diagram	School teams discussed and suggested revisions on poster-size driver diagrams
Closing and reflection	Group reflection on the day and year

those from other schools, rather than engage in the formal disciplined inquiry. The showcase was a success. Teachers excitingly asked each other questions and gained new ideas to try in their classrooms.

The Network's Outcome, End of Year 1

Unlike my previous experience with principals, I deemed this network a success. I began the 2017–2018 school year with a specific evaluation capacity building objective: We would build improvement science capacity and embed processes within the schools. My hope was that by the end of the year, teachers would be able to

- understand and use a driver diagram,

- develop aligned change ideas,

- gather meaningful evidence, and

- engage in inquiry, dialogue, and reflection.

Network teachers demonstrated these improvement science skills and behaviors (although to varying degrees). Three out of the five schools established regular within-school meetings to work on network-related activities. We did have difficulty establishing consistent within-school meetings with Middleview and Marshall due to lack of leadership participation and support as previously discussed.

For our network as a whole, the evidence of successfully building these skills, behaviors, and processes was evident in the number of completed PDSA cycles, a measure of success I had chosen before the network began. The network had completed 63 PDSA cycles between February and May. Of those PDSA cycles, 97% included a change idea that was aligned to the network's theory of practice improvement (i.e., driver diagram.) All the participating teachers, save one, completed at least one PDSA cycle. The number completed by each school is shown in Table 4.5.

While I was primarily interested in building capacity and processes during the inaugural year, it became clear that the intended PDSA learning outcome was occurring, too. Through their PDSA reflections, and observations and interviews, teachers exhibited meaningful and actionable learnings. This new knowledge was generated through the PDSA cycles and by teachers engaging in inquiry and dialogue and sharing with their colleagues, both within their own schools and from other schools. These learnings are discussed more in Chapter 7.

Furthermore, we made progress helping the schools come together as a network. The five schools had a common aim and driver diagram. We had established network routines that fostered teachers engaging in inquiry and dialogue with teachers from other schools. Through these routines, teachers

TABLE 4.5 ● Number of PDSA Cycles Completed			
School	Total number completed	Number of teachers	Average completed per teacher
Roosevelt	22	6	3.67
Marshall	12	6	2.00
Middleview	7	4	1.75
Sawyer	13	4	3.25
Central	9	3	3.00

had the opportunity to hear experiences and perspectives outside of their own school teams and learn new practices and strategies. Teachers also had access to all the completed PDSA forms through our network website. Through our own observations and teacher feedback from network meetings, it was clear that teachers were enjoying the collaboration that occurred within the network.

Although the network demonstrated a positive end-of-year outcome, we still faced challenges. While an average number of PDSAs completed per teachers is reported in Table 4.5 for comparison purposes, there was variation within the number completed by teachers within in a school. For example, and most disparate, one teacher at Central completed seven PDSA cycles, while the other teachers completed one cycle, each. We also struggled to determine common network measures to monitor our improvements. Even though teachers were collecting meaningful data as part of their PDSA cycles, we still needed to develop practical measures aligned to the driver diagram to evaluate whether we were making progress toward our network aim.

Conclusion

The network's narrative demonstrated the importance of balancing rigor to the process and flexibility to meet teachers' needs. To be successful, it was imperative that we provided the space and time to honor our teachers' experiences and learn from them. The next three chapters further examine what facilitated our teachers and schools being prepared to successfully participate in the network. That is, what factors, structures, and/or conditions were needed for schools and individuals to build the improvement science capacity and implement PDSA cycles? And what factors, structures, and/or conditions were needed to generate meaningful individual and school learnings? Chapters 5 and 6 impart findings regarding what helped the University build teachers' and schools' improvement science capacity. Chapter 7 unpacks the networks learnings that were generated and what contributed to them.

Questions for Discussion

1. What narrative examples, if any, resonated with your own experiences leading change?

2. How was the author uncovering and responding to challenges that emerged throughout the process?

3. What rigor versus flexibility decisions have you had to consider in your own contexts or organizations?

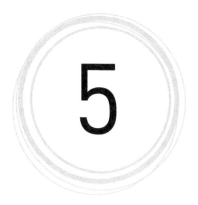

A Tale of Two Visions - Building Individual Capacity

As mentioned previously, a core principle in improvement science is the inclusion of team members with subject knowledge and profound knowledge (how to improve) (Langley et al., 2009). Therefore, as a networked improvement community that was grounded in improvement science principles, this became a fundamental tenet of our network. This point cannot be overstated, as illustrated by what transpired in the early days of the network.

When we started the network, I knew nothing about math instruction and Tom knew little about improvement science and its underlying evaluation concepts. As the network lead, I was responsible for meeting with all our schools, in-between the network convenings. Tom was already responsible for providing math professional development to numerous schools, but the plan was for him to attend most of our school meetings. I presumed the teachers would be able to fill the math subject knowledge void if Tom were unavailable for any reason. My assumption was wrong. The teachers did possess subject knowledge to certain degrees, *but* not the type of math instructional knowledge needed to transform practice.

This became obvious to me during a meeting with Sawyer's teachers in the fall. Tom was sick that day, so I was the sole facilitator. Building on the previous month's network convening, I was facilitating a process map regarding students' lack of prerequisite skills. The math teachers and I were in the school library huddled around a large rectangular table. We mapped out the steps (processes) they currently take when students lack the necessary prerequisite skills for a lesson. When they began brainstorming an ideal process for addressing the problem, the teachers offered ideas including teaching a "Unit Zero" at the start of the school year and teaching the missing skills during lesson warm-ups. Since we were already 4 months into the school year, I directed the conversation around the latter idea. The idea of teaching a lacking prerequisite skill, such as long division, during the warm-up sounded viable and reasonable because I lacked essential subject knowledge. I did not know any better. But Tom did.

Soon after learning Tom's full instructional vision while developing the driver diagram, I realized my deficiency. I not only realized the importance of subject knowledge, particularly when facilitating a conversation such as the one at Sawyer, I saw the need in a new light: It was not merely about content knowledge, but more important about a vision for changing practice that possibly required an outside perspective. Teaching a skill during the lesson warm-up was a contributory learning that could improve an immediate problem, but it was unlikely to transform instructional practice or solve a complex problem. The teachers were brainstorming but only within their current, known instructional paradigm and system. *How would they know a different way to approach instruction, and why would we expect them to?*

In this chapter, I cover:

- The Math Instructional Vision (Subject Knowledge)

- The Vision for Building Improvement Science Capacity (Profound Knowledge)

- The Network's Initial Improvement Science Capacity

- How the Two Visions Intersect

The Math Instructional Vision (Subject Knowledge)

Tom envisioned another way of teaching. His instructional vision was grounded in the National Council of Teachers of Mathematics (NCTM) (2014) report, *Principles to Actions: Ensuring Mathematical Success for All*, and Cognitively Guided Instruction (CGI) principles (Carpenter et al., 1999). CGI is a teacher professional development program that focuses on eliciting, understanding, and building on students' mathematical thinking (Carpenter et al., 1999). One of the principles is to build on what students know and rely on an understanding of students' learning trajectories to make instructional decisions.

As mentioned in the previous chapter, *Principles to Actions: Ensuring Mathematical Success for All* (NCTM, 2014) played a prominent role in the development of our driver diagram. It provided a framework of eight mathematics teaching practices:

1. Establish mathematics goals to focus learning.

2. Implement tasks that promote reasoning and problem solving.

3. Use and connect mathematical representations.

4. Facilitate meaningful mathematical discourse.

5. Pose purposeful questions.

6. Build procedural fluency from conceptual understanding.

7. Support productive struggle in learning mathematics.

8. Elicit and use evidence of student thinking.

Tom's concept of quality math instruction guided the network. At the network convenings, he always kicked off the meeting with a number sense routine, such as "Which One Doesn't Belong," or choral counting. He also thoughtfully prepared problem examples that would apply to grades 6 through 9. He would project the problem on the room screen, and then have the teachers play the role of student. Nimbly moving around the room, Tom would call on them, probing for answers, and pushing them to explain their thinking. His favorite phrase was, "Turn and talk," promoting mathematical discourse among the teachers. Using poster paper, he demonstrated how to easily collect evidence of students' thinking by writing down what was being said, and who said it. Tom also provided opportunities for the teachers to ask questions and reflect on how they would apply these ideas to their own students. All his exercises connected to the mathematical standards and modeled quality instruction in line with his stance, which was projected on one of his slides: Effective teaching of mathematics engages students in solving and discussing tasks that promote mathematical reasoning and problem solving and allow multiple entry points and varied solution strategies (NCTM, p. 12).

The teachers enjoyed this time, often raising their hands and laughing at Tom's jokes. As one teacher exclaimed, "I'd do math all day if we could do this. This is fun!" Another teacher further explained the value in Tom's activities.

> *I think as a math student. Like the math student piece, I've kind of seen how ideas could be presented or taught. That's another thing that I've appreciated . . . is the process that we go through to kind of breakdown how a brain would attack this.*

Philosophically, Tom's instructional viewpoint also connected to equity. When we first started visiting schools together, he often confided his concern when a teacher would offhandedly refer to some of their students as the "low" students or the "high" students. Based on his experiences, he suspected that some of those low students were also former or current English Language Learners. His purpose for introducing number sense routines was not only to elicit student thinking, but also to provide opportunities to shift teacher thinking. He wanted teachers to understand that there are different ways to engage those low students and build on existing student understanding rather than focus on their lacking mathematical skills. To this end, he mindfully shifted conversations during our in-school meetings to discuss PDSA results, commonly asking, "What did you learn about your student's thinking?" and "How can you build on your student's thinking?"

The Vision for Building Improvement Science Capacity (Profound Knowledge)

I also had a vision. As briefly discussed in the previous chapters, my aim for building improvement science capacity during Year 1 centered on teachers' learning processes and embedding them in the schools. I approached this undertaking with an evaluation capacity building lens. The concept of evaluation capacity building is discussed in Chapter 2, but as a reminder it can be succinctly defined as "an intentional process to increase individual motivation, knowledge, and skills, and to enhance a group or organization's ability to conduct or use evaluation" (Labin et al., 2012, p. 308). Evaluation capacity building could focus on all three individual areas: knowledge and understanding, skills and behaviors, and affective or attitudes. Or it could concentrate on one or two areas (Preskill & Boyle, 2008). My primary focus was on teachers building particular skills and behaviors. By the end of the first year, I wanted teachers to demonstrate the following:

- use a driver diagram to develop change ideas that were aligned with the network's theory of practice improvement

- gather meaningful evidence that could be used to evaluate and modify the change idea

- engage in disciplined inquiry with their colleagues using the PDSA format

Improvement science consists of more components—understanding and conducting causal and systems analysis, developing a driver diagram, creating measures to monitor improvements toward the aim—but I differentiated between what I believed teachers could realistically accomplish with limited time and what expertise I needed to provide as the improvement science specialist. While it was certainly possible to impart these technical components to teachers, it did not seem practical. Schools are hectic and chaotic environments. Teachers already have a lot on their plates on a daily basis. In my view, their foremost role in the network was to bring their teaching experiences to the shared problem of practice, experiment with ideas in the classroom, engage in inquiry and dialogue with their colleagues, and reflect on how they can continuously improve. My role was to provide the evaluation expertise, which included facilitating the technical aspects of improvement science.

At this point, it is also important to distinguish the ideas of individual and organizational learning capacity from an evaluation capacity building perspective. My goal was to build both. Individual capacity relates to building participants knowledge, skills, and attitudes (Labin et al., 2012; Preskill & Boyle, 2008). Organizational learning capacity, in the context of evaluation capacity building in schools, refers to whether leadership values learning and the evaluation process and whether the school has a culture of inquiry, has the necessary systems and structures for engaging in the evaluation process, and offers opportunities to access and disseminate evaluation information (Labin et al., 2012; Preskill & Boyle, 2008).

I envisioned developing individual skills and processes and embedding them at an organizational level. This served two purposes: (1) building the skills mentioned previously through consistency and practice, and (2) the transfer of learning to the workplace or mainstreaming to develop a sustainable learning culture in schools. I wanted to build organizational learning habits, so this was my concern in Year 1 rather than actually improving the problem of practice. I recognized that this was an incremental route, and my goal was process oriented. Again, I was playing the long game. We would work with schools, both on-site and at network convenings, so that they would embed processes to continually engage in improvement and evaluative inquiry, even after improving our identified problem of practice. Improvement would not be an "add-on project," but would become a way of working (Rother, 2010).

The Network's Initial Improvement Science Capacity

To gain a sense of the network's initial capacity regarding improvement science, I conducted a survey at the end of our first convening in September. Tables 5.1 and 5.2 show the results for the capacity-related questions for the five case study schools. For the most part, participants (other than Roosevelt) were not familiar with improvement science concepts and tools. Notably, more than half of all participants (14) indicated that they were at least somewhat familiar with process maps, even though later work with the teachers demonstrated that they were unfamiliar with an *improvement science* process map. In this case, the disconnect likely reflected an instance of teachers not knowing what they do not know. *Process map* is a seemingly generic term but has a specific meaning and application in improvement science. In this context, a process map is more technical and includes start and end points, decision points, and open and closed loops. It was clear when working with teachers that they were not familiar with these more technical aspects, even though they understood the basic concept of how one process flowed to another.

TABLE 5.1 ● Teacher and Administrators Familiarity With Improvement Science Concepts						
Before today, how familiar or unfamiliar were you with the following?	I don't know what this is	Not at all familiar	A little familiar	Somewhat familiar	Familiar	Extremely familiar	n
Improvement science	0	10	2	2	5	4	23
Root cause analysis (e.g., 5 Whys)	0	9	2	2	5	5	23
Driver diagrams	1	10	3	4	3	2	23
Process maps	0	4	5	5	5	4	23
PDSA cycles	1	7	2	4	3	6	23
Systems thinking	1	7	1	7	4	3	23

Note: Survey of network participants from the first network convening, September 2017.

Findings of actual unawareness of the more technical aspects of improvement activities existed elsewhere, too. Almost all teachers reported that they were somewhat confident to confident that they could engage in improvement-oriented activities from the outset (Table 5.2). Yet it became clear while working with them that they were, in fact, unaware of specific processes for engaging in these undertakings. For example, as demonstrated by Table 5.1, most teachers were not familiar with root cause analysis, even though all were at least somewhat confident in their ability to identify barriers to student learning in math. This suggests that teachers may perceive they do not need to build the capacity, despite observations of skills and behaviors that demonstrated otherwise.

The challenge of building improvement science capacity among teachers was not merely in helping them value improvement. Most of our network already did value it. On an initial fall survey (not shown), 15 out of the 21 teachers indicated that it was extremely useful to experiment with new teaching practices, when it came to their own teaching. Rather, the challenge here was in demonstrating that the tools and evaluative processes for improving are valuable, too. This proved more difficult.

TABLE 5.2 ● Teacher Confidence in Improvement-Oriented Capacity						
How confident or not confident are you that you can:	Not at all confident	A little confident	Somewhat confident	Confident	Extremely confident	n
Identify potential barriers to students' learning math/alg. concepts?	0	0	8	9	4	21
Make changes to your teaching or classroom practices that could improve student learning in math/alg.?	0	0	4	12	4	20
Test whether a change in your teaching or classroom practices resulted in an improvement of your practice?	0	3	7	8	3	21
Collect meaningful data to evaluate whether a change in your teaching or classroom practices resulted in an improvement of your practice?	0	1	6	12	2	21

(*Continued*)

TABLE 5.2 ● (Continued)						
Analyze data to evaluate whether a change in your teaching or classroom practices resulted in an improvement of your practice?	1	1	7	9	3	21

Note. Survey of network participants from the first network convening, September 2017. Teachers only.

Throughout this first year, more than one teacher initially resisted conducting the PDSA cycle. They insisted that they already did the same process in their practices (without formally documenting it). While we did not challenge whether this was true, we did respond by reminding them that the network was a collaborative endeavor. Its purpose was not only about individual learning, but documenting their experimentation and reflection provided an opportunity for others to learn from them. They never argued this point, which suggested that our teachers valued collaboration with their colleagues.

This notion was apparent and reinforced throughout the entire school year. On the initial fall survey, the teachers indicated that it was useful to collaborate with other teachers to reflect on improving practices; with 17 out of 21 teachers responding that it was extremely useful (not shown). Feedback from network convenings frequently showed that teachers appreciated the time to work with department teams and to talk with teachers from other schools. Interviewed teachers also expressed this sentiment. When asked what stood out for them about the network, the most common answer was collaboration with other teachers.

The Two Visions Intersect

Our team found one way to engage teachers in learning improvement science skills, even if they were not interested in the tools and processes, was by learning in context. While this was not an overt strategy when we started this network, it became apparent that teachers were more motivated to improve math instructional practice rather than improve their ability to improve. Put another way, most teachers did not demonstrate a desire to get better at driver diagrams or PDSAs cycles. They expressed a desire to be better at their instructional practices to help their students. One teacher expressed this sentiment by comparing the early large network meetings that did not include math instructional professional development to the later small network meetings that did. She explained:

> Yeah, I guess the one negative thing from the beginning of the year, it was just the [large network] days that were like, full days, and not feeling like, it was moving very fast . . . But more recent things of, you know, seeing and working with more specific ways of adjusting to meet our students' needs. That has felt more helpful. And I know that there had to be, there had to be big picture conversation of like, "What's actually going on? Let's not just like, fix a problem the way that all the books say we should fix the problem." Um, it just felt like, it took a little while to get authentic.

This teacher was communicating that building capacity (problem solving) in the context of adjusting to their students' needs felt more authentic than learning improvement science in the abstract with an undefined problem of practice. In doing so, she acknowledged the value of placing learning in the day-to-day teacher context, not just an educational context.

Although we had not formally drawn on situated cognition learning theory during Year 1, it is apparent on reflection that we were subscribing to its principles (Brown et al., 1989; Merriam & Bierema, 2014). Over the years, numerous people have told me they find improvement science to be overly abstract and "jargon-y." Situating the improvement science language and concepts into the everyday work of the teacher's classroom provided a way for teachers to construct meaning of these abstract concepts.

Evaluation capacity building theory also recognizes a need for situating evaluation activities in participants' workplace context. Preskill and Boyle's (2008) multidisciplinary model incorporates adult and workplace learning theories and explicitly connects sustainable evaluation practice to the capacity-building activities through the "transfer of knowledge." Transfer of knowledge refers to the idea of skills and concepts learned in one setting being applied to another (i.e., the workplace) (Preskill & Boyle, 2008). Furthermore, they assert that it is crucial to create transfer of learning opportunities throughout the capacity-building initiative. Those leading these endeavors should consider how to foster knowledge transfer to the workplace when determining learning strategies and objectives, communicating expectations about implementing, and evaluating their own capacity-building efforts (Preskill & Boyle, 2008).

The ability of teachers to make sense of the evaluative concepts in their own contexts was evident at our April network convening. They were asked to explain why they believed their latest change idea would improve the network's global aim (i.e., engage all students and meet their variety of learning needs). We requested they use the driver diagram to illustrate their thoughts. One-by-one, teachers from each of the schools stood up at their tables while other team members held the driver diagram. They articulated how their idea was connected to a particular secondary driver then connected to one of the primary drivers, which would then improve student learning. We (University hub) were thrilled, if not a little astonished, that they had effortlessly described their theory of improvement *and* used the language of improvement science (i.e., change idea, secondary driver, primary driver, aim). This successful moment was the result of the two visions intersecting.

Another instance of the two parallel learning tracks—building improvement science skills and improving math instruction to engage all students and meet their variety of learning needs—fruitfully intersecting was the PDSA cycle. At the January network convening, we introduced Tom's number sense routines, specifically the Which One Doesn't Belong routine, and the PDSA process. Which One Doesn't Belong is a mathematical reasoning task where teachers project four quadrants, with pictures or numeric expressions or equations for example, and then ask students which one of these doesn't belong and why. The task can be used in different courses and customized with the appropriate mathematical content. We were deliberate about teaching them both the mathematical routine and the PDSA cycle in the same meeting, again drawing on the evaluation capacity building concept of transferring knowledge. Although we did not specify that teachers should try the number sense routine as their change idea, the routine modeled the type of activity they should be experimenting with in their PDSA. For example, Which One Doesn't Belong was:

- Quick to implement: Teachers could experiment with it the next week without requiring a lot of planning time. It also only required about 15–20 minutes of class time. Teachers could complete a full PDSA cycle within a week since it could be tested during one class.

- Manageable: Teachers only needed slides with the four images or mathematical terms (which did require some planning time). Tom modeled how to lead the activity. He also demonstrated how to easily collect data for the PDSA cycle by writing down what was said, and who said it, during the activity. This was practical data collection: It informed instruction and assessed the level of student engagement in the activity.

- Meaningful: The activity was aligned to the network's aim—engaging all students in mathematical activities. It could also initiate meaningful reflection as to which students participated in the activity and why and what assumptions teachers made.

Most teachers chose the Which One Doesn't Belong activity for their first PDSA, and we were amenable with that choice. Not only was the activity in line with Tom's vision, but it also helped scaffold learning the PDSA process. We felt this was crucial. Teachers were not charged with identifying an instructionally appropriate change idea to try in their classroom, mastering how to implement it quickly, *and* learning a whole new process for evaluating that change. Our priority was for them to learn this process rather than innovate change ideas.

The PDSA structure facilitated the math instructional learning, too. Essentially, the PDSA cycle is a form of adult experiential learning (Langley et al., 2009; Merriam & Bierema, 2014). Experiential learning refers to learning through life or workplace experiences and the reflection on those experiences (Dewey, 1963; Merriam & Bierema, 2014). Because many teachers opted to try Tom's number sense routines, the PDSA cycle provided a structure for putting that professional development into practice. The process itself required that teachers experience the number sense routine in practice (Do) and then reflect on that experience (Study).

One teacher illustrated how PDSA cycles contributed to her instructional learning. In this example, the tool she is testing through the PDSA process is the Which One Doesn't Belong activity:

Every single time there [were] at least two things going on, it would be the actual tool that I was testing. And so, maybe I was testing Which One Doesn't Belong. But not only was I testing the tool, I was also testing the concept I was putting in the tool. And that's kind of why I was saying it'd be nice to have some examples, because sometimes if I didn't choose a great concept to place in the tool, then it would die. But then, if I did it in a way that made sense to the kids and made sense to what we were doing, like, the tool worked. So I think that's what it is. It made me think how to best use the tool. And if something didn't work, it was usually not the tool. It was usually what I put in it.

From this example, it is also clear how the process not only led the teacher to consider the tool or activity, but also reconsider her decisions about how to use the tool. As discussed in Chapter 7, learning can also be transformative when the experience and reflection leads to the questioning of assumptions and reconsidering how instruction occurs rather than merely incremental improvement to the current instructional practices (Argyris & Schön, 1996; Merriam & Bierema, 2014).

Conclusion

Tom's notion of quality mathematical instruction and my plan for building improvement science capacity were more than complementary, they were synergistic. Even though we had not explicitly discussed how the two visions were intertwined during the first year, they guided our decisions every step of the way. His mathematical instruction expertise advanced our ability to build improvement science skills by providing context and an incentive to build evaluative capacity. This chapter illuminates the significance of establishing visions in both the content area (subject knowledge) and improvement science capacity (profound knowledge) and for the experts in both areas to deliberately work together. After walking out of a PDSA meeting at one of our schools, Tom and I joked that we were "in each other's head." Throughout the meeting, I had asked teachers, "What did you learn about your students thinking?" and he had asked, "What is your evidence?"

Questions for Discussion

1. Why was it important for the author and Tom to: (1) Each establish their own vision? (2) Bring the two visions together?

2. What are your own experiences either teaching or learning technical research or evaluation-related concepts? How might teaching and/or learning them within the context of life or work experiences further the capacity to implement them?

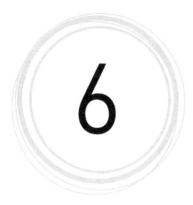

The Importance of Being Structured - Building Organizational Capacity

There is a Central Law of Improvement that states, "Every system is perfectly designed to deliver the results it produces" (Langley et al., 2009, p. 79). In Chapter 2, I discussed this idea in the context of complexity science and the espoused system purpose versus its actual designed purpose, whether intentional or unintentional. In this chapter, I offer this concept in the context of change initiative work structures. If you do not set up structures to do the work, the work will not occur. Herein lies the potential irony of improvement science in education. In my experience, I have seen and participated in improvement science initiatives where educators from multiple schools were assembled, taught improvement science concepts and tools, urged to apply them at their schools, and then released. The folks in charge of these convenings (including me) sent educators off without attending to the work structures in their schools, instead hoping with fingers crossed that teachers and administrators would make the time and effort to follow through on their improvement science promises.

For me, the most obvious example of the unkept promise is the Plan, Do, Study, Act (PDSA) cycle. While learning about networked improvement communities, I attended a network convening of another network, which had been in existence for a couple years. During the meeting, I noticed there was no mention of the PDSA cycle. I asked the organizer about it, and she indicated they struggled to implement them. I then asked whether they worked with teachers at their schools. She replied they did not. This was reminiscent of my previous experience where it was challenging for principals to implement regular PDSA cycles. We hoped to inspire, motivate, and build capacity at central meetings, with little attention paid to their existing work structures back at the schools. In that case, we did not want to dictate how principals applied the process at their sites. We felt that was their purview, not ours. However, schools are hectic environments where teachers' and administrators' time and energy are forever being pulled in different directions. The project failed to gain traction and resulted in no actionable learnings. Our system proved it was perfectly designed to achieve the insufficient results that it did.

In this chapter, I cover:

- Organizational Capacity

- Individual Versus Organizational Capacity

- Network Structures

Organizational Capacity

The previous chapter briefly discussed the purpose of embedding improvement science processes within schools as part of individual and organizational evaluation capacity building goals. This chapter expands on the findings related to those ideas, particularly in terms of the organizational learning conditions necessary to support capacity building and continuous improvement. Preskill & Boyle (2008) refer to organizational learning capacity as "an organization's culture, leadership, systems and structures, and communications that support and encourage organizational learning" (p. 453). Furthermore, they also acknowledge that it can be difficult for evaluation to become rooted in an organization due to continual contextual changes (e.g., staff turnover). Their concepts and ideas resonated with our experiences. Schools are complex social systems. Actors are always adapting and responding to contextual changes. Therefore, building and sustaining improvement science practices requires the "development of systems, processes, policies, and plans that help embed evaluation work into the way the organization" works (Preskill & Boyle, 2008, p. 444).

School Structures

Our ability to regularly meet with schools and build systems and structures was related to their preexisting organizational capacity, particularly in the form of leadership. From the outset, our University team shared our expectation of holding regular, on-site meetings with the teachers and administrators (except in the case at Middleview as previously discussed). But working at the schools required time and space, both contingent on the commitment of administrator leadership to provide them. That was one of the most significant roles administrators played.

In Year 1, we encountered differences among the schools' leadership that impacted our ability to build in-school work structures. I found this to be connected to the teachers' ability to develop their individual improvement science capacity. Table 6.1 shows how the number of in-school meetings corresponds with the number of completed PDSA cycles by school.

For example, the principal at Central exhibited a high level of commitment by carving out time during the school day for his three teachers, every 2 weeks. Teachers met during a conference period, even though they all had different class schedules and free periods. The principal found coverage for the teachers and alternated periods to lessen his teachers' burden. The administrators at Sawyer also prioritized our meeting time with schedule accommodations. Teachers were released early, 1 day a week for professional development time. That gave us time to work with their teachers at least once a month.

The Roosevelt administrator also supported our work with her teachers, but their situation was unique. Because they already had improvement science experience and meeting structures for discussing PDSAs cycles we did not organize their within-school work structures. Instead, we attended their existing meetings as participants rather than as facilitators so that we did not interfere with their existing processes. However, there was a facilitator (their lead teacher) and I did interject at times to coach the use of improvement science tools and methods.

As discussed previously in Chapter 3 we had difficulty scheduling regular meetings at Marshall. Their administrator wanted more flexibility with the process than other principals and provided little assistance with Samantha's request to establish a set time to work with his teachers. Only through Samantha's persistence we were able to schedule meetings, but they were inconsistent and never became part of a regular schedule. The absence of a set meeting time adversely impacted the number of times that we met with them.

Middleview was another exception, but only because we did not place expectations on them due to our own assumptions regarding their ability to commit time and energy (as discussed in Chapter 3). We did not meet with the principal at the beginning of the year, thus, he never committed to carving out time and space for us. Once Middleview built their math team by mid-year, we attempted to organize time directly with the teachers. They were already

TABLE 6.1 ● Number of PDSA Cycles Completed and In-School Meetings			
School	Total number completed	Average completed per teacher	Number of times we met with them
Roosevelt	22	3.67	5
Marshall	12	2.00	4
Middleview	7	1.75	1
Sawyer	13	3.25	8
Central	9	3.00	8

Note: Roosevelt already had preexisting improvement science capacity and PDSA meeting structures.

having weekly, after-school meetings for another continuous improvement process championed by the district, so they tried to append our network to that recurring meeting. We attempted this several times, and each time, we were only given an average of 15 to 20 minutes, which proved to be insufficient. It was a challenge to make our brief time together meaningfully productive. We did, however, meet with them for one 2-hour session as a *make up* for missing a network convening.

Facilitating Collaboration Conducive to Improvement

Providing time and space for collaboration, while a crucial first step, does not ensure that the collaboration will be productive and/or promote learnings needed to solve complex problems of practice. At the very least, collaboration time should have a commonality of purpose and promote dialogue and discussion. At its best, collaboration advances team learning through the alignment of its members, whereby insights are generated and put into action (Senge, 2006). Through the initial fall survey, network members were asked about what routines, meetings, and other structures their school already had in place for teachers to collaborate toward improving their teaching practices. Almost all teachers (90%, 19 out of 21) indicated that they had collaboration time through some type of regular meeting (e.g., department meeting), common conference period, and/or professional development time (not shown). However, in that same survey, only about half the teachers and administrators (48%, 10 out of 21) indicated that they met at least monthly, on average, with other teachers to discuss what helps students learn best (not shown). Additionally, less than a third of network teachers (28%, 5 out of 18) said that they asked another teacher for help or feedback on their own teaching practices at least once a month, on average (not shown). These data suggest that although teachers already met regularly, much their time was spent working together on topics other than improving student learning and/ or their own practices.

Furthermore, I found that when they did meet regarding how to improve student learning and instructional practices, the structures were not always conducive to dialogue, discussion, and/or inquiry. An observation at Roosevelt illustrates this example. I attended one of their math department meetings where they discussed PDSA cycles. The lead teacher facilitated this meeting. She was extremely structured. Teachers were given a set amount of time (e.g., 10 minutes) to share what they tried in their classroom and their results. Teachers sat in a circle and took turns speaking. After a while, I noticed that the teachers were not asking each other questions. I asked a few questions in an attempt to start a dialogue, but the lead teacher requested that we hold our questions until the end, after everyone had shared. I surmised that she was extremely concerned about keeping to the schedule and not going over the meeting time allotted. I was acutely aware that teachers' time is a finite commodity, so this was understandable, but it was also a conundrum that thwarted the ability to engage in productive inquiry and dialogue. By the end of that meeting, very little teacher-to-teacher questioning had occurred, rather it was teachers individually sharing before moving on to the next person.

Participatory, collaborative, and more specifically evaluative inquiry are social practices that requires organization members (i.e., teachers) to dialogue, reflect, ask each other questions, and continually identify and clarify values, beliefs, and assumptions (Preskill & Torres, 1999). Evaluative inquiry is analogous to the type of inquiry expected in improvement science endeavors. Members, ideally with multiple perspectives, engage in continuous organizational learning to investigate and address issues related to organizational processes and outcomes. A crucial and necessary component of evaluative inquiry is dialogue through which team members connect, ask questions, develop shared understandings around complex issues, and surface assumptions (Preskill & Torres, 1999). The evaluator's primary role is to be a facilitator, and as such, may train participants in dialogue skills to build their inquiry capacity. Because of our experience at Roosevelt, along with other similar experiences, we taught the teachers how to engage in inquiry and dialogue (as discussed in Chapter 4) in an effort to cultivate team learning. We encouraged them to use the protocol that we developed for network PDSA sessions in their in-school discussions, too. Our hope was not that they use a protocol every time they engaged in dialogue and inquiry but would eventually develop a routine for asking meaningful questions (i.e., to push each other's thinking). While teachers did not always follow the protocol during school PDSA meetings, I did observe an increase in questioning, particularly at Roosevelt.

On the opposite end of the structure, I observed how collaboration time can be too unstructured to promote constructive dialogue. As a teacher from another school shared: "It's always a struggle to collaborate without turning it into a bitch session . . . I think we have a pretty positive math department, but at the same time, it does seem like, given time, that's the path we go down."

One of the benefits of improvement science is the provision for structured collaboration around a common purpose. Tools such as a fishbone diagram or a process map organize conversations around potential causes of a problem. These tools can focus the group's dialogue. The driver diagram categorizes thinking around how to improve a problem. The PDSA cycle is a structured format for experimenting and reflecting on results. These tools are helpful for guiding conversations and keeping them on track. As one administrator stated, "I've appreciated just the different systems you've gone through to kind of organize teachers and their thinking, from an outside perspective."

The Benefit of an Outside Facilitator

Our facilitation at in-school meetings served multiple purposes: supporting the use of the improvement science tools, supporting productive collaboration and dialogue, and providing an outside perspective. As mentioned, a key component of our improvement science capacity building vision was the need for an improvement science specialist to facilitate these meetings. (Roosevelt was the exception because they already had existing capacity and desire to lead these meetings.)

In interviews, I asked teachers and administrators whether they would have been comfortable facilitating the in-school meetings, when we developed fishbone diagrams and early pieces of the driver diagrams. Many teachers acknowledged that they did not have the capacity, time, or desire to lead those early meetings. One teacher said it would be like "the blind leading the blind." Another teacher acknowledged the two issues of capacity and burdening a teacher with the responsibility.

> *I don't know if we know enough about it. We've been through it. I don't think we have time, to be perfectly honest. I mean we're running all the time. So that would be an extra burden for someone to go back and research and review, take the time to do this, and just to set it up.*

Even a teacher who felt that she had a solid understanding of the tools indicated that she would not want to add another responsibility to her plate.

> *So, in that sense, it sounds like another responsibility. So, could I show up to a meeting and roll something out? Probably, but if I was supposed to be really thinking about it away from that time, I don't think that's really realistic.*

We also conducted a survey at the end of Year 1 to gauge teachers' ability to lead and facilitate meetings after learning improvement science concepts. The results are shown in Table 6.2. Many teachers felt that they could apply improvement ideas and tools without the help of a facilitator. However, what is especially notable here is that almost none of the teachers (including many of the Roosevelt teachers) indicated that they could teach the concepts to facilitate other teachers within their school teams. The importance of this distinction cannot be overstated. Taken together with the interview results, a common notion arises. For the most part, teachers did not feel they have the capacity to teach and facilitate other teachers around the use of improvement science tools, nor did they want the responsibility. Even those who perceived that they have the capacity, acknowledged that it is more efficient and less burdensome to have an outside expert lead the meeting. Preskill and Boyle (2008) acknowledge the importance of the facilitator in their multidisciplinary evaluation capacity building model. They purport that the facilitator's expertise, as well as their knowledge of the organization and its members, can influence how and to what extent participants build evaluation capacity. This idea is further supported by other networks who have found an improvement science facilitator to be beneficial as well (Proger et al., 2017).

TABLE 6.2 ● Teacher Self Ratings of Knowledge and Skills of Improvement Science Concepts, Terms, and Tools

How would you rate your level of knowledge and skills for the following concepts, terms, or tools?	I don't know what this is	I can recall this concept, term, or tool	I understand this and how it connects to our work	I can apply this with assistance from Univ. facilitator	I can apply this without assistance from Univ. facilitator	I can teach this to facilitate and lead our school team	n
Conducting root cause analysis (e.g., Fishbone Diagram, 5 Whys)	0	0	0	8	8	1	17
Using a process map	1	0	2	8	6	0	17
Developing a driver diagram	0	0	1	6	9	0	16
Developing a change idea aligned to the driver diagram	0	0	1	3	10	2	16
Conducting a Plan–Do–Study–Act (PDSA) cycle	0	0	0	3	12	2	17
Collecting PDSA data/evidence to inform whether the change idea resulted in an improvement	0	1	1	0	13	2	17
Developing meaningful process measures	1	1	2	3	9	1	17
Developing meaningful outcome measures	1	1	2	3	8	2	17

Note: Survey of network participants from the last network convening. May 2017.

Furthermore, the presence of network facilitators at the in-school meetings helped teachers feel supported throughout this process. As one teacher enthusiastically described,

> *That's one of the things I've been, like, telling my colleagues, especially the ones coming into Algebra 1. . . . I'm like, "Dude, they come and work with us during the meetings to prepare us for our next meeting," which is awesome because then it becomes productive time, you know?*

Facilitating the meetings also provided an opportunity for an outside perspective during these activities. Not only did it provide an instructional perspective outside their current paradigm, as discussed in Chapter 5, but also it provided a more objective viewpoint that assisted in propelling the work forward. One teacher highlighted an example, "I mean, I think at one point in one of those, we had, like, four different Post-Its for the same thing. And you guys were able to guide this. 'Maybe you guys could put this together.' 'Oh, cool!'"

Collaboration Around Instructional Practices

The evidence suggests that teachers were engaging in more improvement-oriented collaboration and dialogue around their practices by the end of Year 1. The end-of-year survey indicated that a greater proportion of teachers were partaking in collaboration with other teachers around improving student learning and their own teacher practices. Almost three out of four (71%, 12 out of 17) said that they met at least monthly, on average, with other teachers to discuss what helps students learn best (not shown). Now, more than half of the teachers (57%, 8 out of 14) indicated that they asked another teacher for help or feedback on their own teaching practices at least once a month on average (not shown).[1]

These results, combined with observation and interview data, suggest that regular in-school meetings structured around improvement activities such as PDSA cycles were leading to more discussions about student learning and instructional practices. As Tom noticed, the frequency with which teachers were meeting and reflecting was shifting conversations and thinking more toward how best to engage students in mathematical learning. He noted:

> *What's also really, really structured is the consistency by which teachers are given time to think about their practice and come to the table to reflect about their practice, and to share some of the things that they've come to learn. That, I think, has been paramount to shifting the needle a little bit for some of the teachers with regards to their instruction and thinking about how the kids are engaging with mathematics. And I know that because I previously worked with*

---

[1]Caution should be used if directly comparing to results of the first survey. Not all the participants were the same in both surveys.

folks at Middleview and Sawyer, and I know that in my time, definitely at Sawyer, it had been really challenging to get momentum, to build momentum. And I feel like the consistency by which we are meeting with them has been very much conducive to them, again, thinking about their practice, thinking about how they've been engaging kids, or how their students are engaging with the mathematics.

Consistency

In *Toyota Kata*, Rother (2010) explains that a continually improving organization is one that builds thinking and behavior patterns and systematic routines for adapting and improving. When employees practice these patterns and routines as part of their day-to-day work, they have the means and habits for improving desired outcomes. Rother (2010) acknowledges that the challenge is developing and maintaining these routines. Preskill and Boyle (2008) also assert the importance of providing opportunities for participants to practice their learning when building evaluation capacity.

Thus, not surprisingly, I found that consistency and practice were key. By regularly working with the schools, we were not only trying to build improvement science skills, but we were also trying to develop habits and routines, both individual and organizational. During interviews, many teachers expressed that they learned some process, such as the driver diagram, by continually using it or revisiting the tool. Another example is the protocol that we developed to assist teachers with engaging in productive inquiry and dialogue, as discussed previously. Meeting observations indicated that teachers were becoming more comfortable asking probing questions and sharing their thoughts. While some of this comfort might have been related to practice using tools and the protocol, it could also be due to simply spending more time with their colleagues in this forum. Either way, it was the consistency of these meetings that contributed to behavior changes.

Regular meetings with schools also helped the University support network schools. Because we met with the teachers frequently, we built relationships with them, which then contributed to them sharing honest feedback with us. As discussed in earlier chapters, some teachers pushed back on conducting PDSA cycles during state testing, documenting reflections, or were upfront about why they did not complete the run chart pilot activity. We had these conversations when meeting with schools between network convenings, which allowed us to uncover and respond to emergent challenges when planning the next network meeting. Even when concerns were not explicitly stated to us, we detected potential issues during our attendance. For example, as illustrated previously, it was during school meetings that I discerned that teachers at some schools were not asking each other questions, or time constraints (e.g., a 60-minute department meeting) were limiting productive inquiry and dialogue.

Rother (2010) offered a definition of continuous improvement that we, the hub, pursued in our work of leading the network that instructs "moving towards a desired state through an unclear territory by being sensitive to and responding to actual conditions on the ground" (p. 43). It was only through regular meetings with teachers that we were aware of actual conditions on the ground. Only then could we strive to continually improve our own processes for preparing schools to successfully participate in the network.

Consistency was beneficial to the network in other ways, too. It was through in-school meetings that we were able to develop a driver diagram that reflected each school's concerns. We heard their discussions and compiled their causal analysis artifacts. Rather than trying to bring five schools together to reach agreement, we more efficiently served as the consensus makers.

Individual Versus Organizational Capacity

The importance of building organizational capacity and consistent work structures cannot be overstated. However, while embedding work structures and systems in the schools contributed to teachers' ability to implement PDSA cycles and successfully participate in the network, their preexisting individual capacity was a factor, too. This point is demonstrated by the variation in PDSA cycle completion among teachers within the same school.

There were noticeable differences between the teachers who completed the most PDSA cycles within their school and those who completed the fewest. Interviews with teachers who completed fewer PDSA cycles suggested that they were more concerned with classroom management and discipline than the other teachers. These teachers also tended to be more teacher-directed in their instructional style. That is, they preferred leading the instruction in the classrooms rather than students directing their own learning through collaborative groups. On the other hand, teachers who completed more PDSA cycles reported that they were comfortable experimenting with new ideas in their classroom, and already *informally* reflected on their lessons, to tweak and improve them. Thus, these teachers possessed some existing capacity necessary for successful PDSA cycles.

Network Structures

While this chapter emphasizes school organizational structures, it is important to note that network convening structures also contributed to the successful completion of PDSA cycles. For example, we ensured the consistent use of the driver diagram by incorporating it into meeting activities. Our meetings were intentionally structured to provide improvement science and math instructional professional development and/or activities in the morning, and school teamwork time in the afternoon. It was during this afternoon time that teachers would plan their next PDSA cycle. As the year progressed, we began prioritizing this PDSA work time over other convening activities if we did not have time for both. We also started giving them time to complete their individual reflection section of the PSDA form. Through conversations with teachers, it became clear that teachers had difficulty finding the time to reflect and document their thoughts and learning after experimenting in their classroom. When teachers indicated that they were overwhelmed during state testing time, our offer to provide this extra work time assuaged some of their scheduling concerns.

Conclusion

These findings suggest that any hope of developing improvement science capacity of educators, teachers in particular, first requires cooperative in-school work structures. Network leaders substantially benefit from the support of school administrators because they provide the key ingredients: time, space, and necessary supports for teachers. Without these, it is unrealistic to expect teachers to each find the time to prepare and regularly gather in a room with other teachers to facilitate improvement science activities on their own. And to expect them to do so, without any preexisting knowledge and skills, is impractical.

As with building and embedding any new behaviors in an organization, I found that consistency was as crucial as leadership support. Regular and frequent meetings with schools also benefited the hub by providing ongoing opportunities to assess challenges as they arise, acknowledge teacher perspectives and address their concerns. While this chapter highlights the benefits of establishing structures, it is also important to note that embedding these routines within schools is challenging, and it is still a work in progress for our network.

Questions for Discussion

1. What are your experiences engaging in a *collaborative* process with the intent of fostering a change or improvement? What helped facilitate collaboration and progress toward your objective? What challenges did you face?

2. What are your experiences attending meetings that you would deem productive or unproductive? Were there differences in how these meetings were facilitated and structured?

Not All Learning Is Created Equal - Fostering Transformational Organizational Learning

The previous chapters discussed the network hub's goal of building and embedding improvement science skills by the end of Year 1, as demonstrated by the completion of Plan, Do, Study, Act (PDSA) cycles. However, PDSA cycles are only a means to an end. Ultimately, the purpose of improvement science (or any continuous learning process) is to generate collective learnings that can improve complex problems. Therefore, it was also important to consider what learnings were generated during Year 1 and how they were generated.

In this chapter, I cover:

- The Learnings Generated During Year 1

- The Importance of Reflective Structures for Single- and Double-Loop Learning

- Intentionally Designing Activities to Foster Double-Loop Learning

Argyris and Schön's (1996) single-loop and double-loop learning provide a useful way for conceptualizing learning that leads to change. Single-loop learnings are instrumental learnings that lead to improved performance without changing underlying values, norms, or strategies regarding current practices (Argyris & Schön, 1996). Double-loop learnings question underlying values, norms, or strategies, ultimately leading to changes in how and/or why certain practices are being done (Argyris & Schön, 1996). Both types of learning are valuable. Single-loop learning is useful for improving on current practices while double-loop learning is helpful for reconsidering and transforming practice.

Consider the meeting with Sawyer's teachers discussed in Chapter 5. The teachers were working on the challenge surrounding students lacking a prerequisite skill necessary for a lesson, such as long division. During their brainstorming, they devised a solution around teaching prerequisite skills before the lesson as a warm-up. This type of learning through the collaborative dialogue of the teachers is an example of single-loop learning. However, while teaching long division during a warm-up might correct the issue, it does not address the fundamental problem: Incoming students do not know long division. Therefore, the complex problem—a lack of prerequisite skills—will likely persist. In this example, double-loop learning could result from inquiry around how they teach long division in the math classes and questioning their own assumptions regarding how students learn. Teachers would reconsider their own pedagogy and be open to new instructional approaches.

Double loop-learning occurs when the inquiry leads to changes in individual or organizational values of "theories-in-use," defined as patterns that are implicit in individual or organizational behaviors (Argyris & Schön, 1996). Theories-in-use can be compared to "espoused theory" which represents the strategies and values that individuals or organizations advance to explain their actions (Argyris & Schön, 1996). Fundamentally, espoused theory represents the notion of "what we say we do" which can be compared to theories-in-use that signifies "what we actually do" (Senge, 2006).

The ideas of espoused theory and theories-in-use are especially germane to the challenges faced in education. In my experience working with teachers, I have seen espoused theories and theories-in-use in conflict, sometimes unknowingly to the teacher. For example, in our network, one teacher espoused her beliefs that all her students were capable of learning, and she seemed to truly believe it. Yet when she spoke about her students in the meetings, she often referred to them as the "low" students and the "high" students; thus, unwittingly labeling students' ability to learn. In other instances, teachers were more overt about this conflict. They would agree with the school's espoused theory during meetings—that all students can learn math—but also blame their students for a lack of engagement in math rather than acknowledging their own role. Double-loop learning occurs when teachers become aware of these conflicting values and assumptions and resolve them in way that changes their underlying theories-of-use.

These ideas of single-loop and double-loop learning and espoused theory and theories-in-use came to guide many of our network inquiry activities. While we wanted to foster both single- and double-loop learning, we realized that transforming teachers' instructional practices would absolutely require double-loop learning. Single-loop learning on its own would not be enough.

Teachers needed to reconsider how and why they taught certain ways, and not just incrementally improve strategies that fit into their existing paradigm of teaching. As we recognized the need for double-loop learning to solve our complex problem of practice—our current practices are not aligned with students' learning needs today—we attempted to foster it through inquiry structures and activities.

The Learnings Generated During Year 1

The PDSA forms provided evidence of what teachers learned throughout the year. Combining these data with interviews, observations, and the end-of-year survey painted a picture of the type of learning that occurred during Year 1. Incremental learning occurred through the PDSA cycle: Teachers chose a change idea, such as Which One Doesn't Belong, made a prediction, collected data, assessed whether they met the prediction, and through reflection and inquiry, corrected the change idea until it achieved the results they desired. This initial type of learning, one PDSA at a time, was more consistent with single-loop learning. However, through the course of math instructional professional development, PDSA cycles, inquiry and dialogue, and opportunities for reflection, it appeared that some double-loop learning was occurring as well. In these cases, teachers appeared to be shifting their underlying values and assumptions about how their students learn math.

Illustrations of Single-Loop Learning

As part of the PDSA cycles, teachers were asked to reflect on their experimentation of their change idea, including their results, what they learned, and what they will do next. For the purposes of this research, single-loop learnings would be knowledge generated that improved on a practice or strategy, but did not alter underlying assumptions, values, and norms of teachers' practices. I assumed that teachers conducted their PDSA cycles within their existing instructional paradigm because the change ideas were inserted into their current ways of teaching (i.e., adding Which One Doesn't Belong as a warm-up activity). (As described more in the next section, multiple iterations of single-loop learning could lead to double-loop learning when teachers begin to question current practices through the knowledge gained in PDSA cycles, although it is not a necessary precursor.)

Not all teachers provided evidence of single-loop learning in their PDSA forms such as identifying actionable next steps to improve on a strategy or completing multiple iterations that improved on a strategy or current practice. In these cases, for the purposes of this research, I would not classify single-loop learning as occurring because there was no evidence they generated learnings that could improve their instructional performance (regardless of whether it leads to double-loop learning). However, it is quite possible that learnings were still generated and acted on, but not documented. Of the 23 teachers,

16 demonstrated single-loop learnings through their PDSA forms. Differences among teachers tended to be related to the individual and organizational capacity (or lack thereof) needed to complete PDSA cycles, as discussed in previous chapters.

There were many instances of single-loop learning in the network. Figures 7.1 and 7.2 provide examples that exemplify how this learning occurred through the PDSA process. In Figure 7.1, the algebra teacher was building on her first PDSA cycle (not shown) where she tried the Which One Doesn't Below activity during one of her periods. During that class, she incorporated the task as part of her lesson on two-variable association in scatterplots. She predicted that most of her students would engage in the discussion by raising their hands and sharing answers with the whole class. She found that even though more students were participating, compared to previous lessons, there was still unbalanced participation: Some students were not engaged at all, while other students were repeatedly contributing.

Through the second PDSA iteration, Figure 7.1, she improved on the first cycle by having students work in teams, write down their answers and then share by team. This time, she tried the activity in all her algebra periods. Using the data she gathered in the first PSDA cycle, she made incremental adjustments regarding opportunities for students to engage in the activity: volunteering as part of the whole group discussion versus writing first and sharing by team. She also paired the activity more closely with the lesson in this iteration. She indicated that she wanted to continue finding ways to incorporate as a landmark before and after the lesson.

This teacher's experience serves as illustration of valuable single-loop learning. She used data from the first PDSA cycle to modify her approach for providing students opportunities to engage in the activity. Every student engaged this time, at least through writing, and each team shared. She corrected the problem of unbalanced participation among her students. The PDSA learnings fit within her current instructional paradigm. The change was an add-on to her existing lesson rather than altering her underlying values and norms of instruction. In her reflection though, she does express a desire to incorporate more, but at this point, she is only considering incorporating as an activity before or after her usual lessons.

In the next example, a sixth-grade teacher was also building on a previous Which One Doesn't Belong PDSA cycle (not shown). He experimented with the idea in a fraction-related lesson in the last 10 minutes of one of his classes. He predicted that the students would engage in the activity and demonstrate academic vocabulary related to relevant mathematical concepts. He found that while students were engaged in the activity and demonstrated knowledge around fractions, they struggled with reasoning and explaining their ideas. He felt that the use of visuals would further improve students' engagement in the activity and help them articulate their reasoning. Additionally, he thought that visuals would help students better understand the relationship between fractions and whole numbers.

FIGURE 7.1 ● Second PDSA Iteration for Central Teacher, From February 16–23, 2018

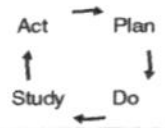

Act → Plan
↑   ↓ Do
Study ←

PDSA CYCLE FORM

Change Idea	Describe: Which One Doesn't Belong for Exponential Functions What is the change: Building on the WODB structure from last time: improve wait time, all students thinking/writing, have teams share in turns before the same people can share again, and preselect some student responses.
Predictions: What improvement do we think will happen?	Like last time, students will have fun and some will share who usually don't. This time, I aim to get even broader participation and more students' voices. I also want to highlight when students build on something a classmate shared.
Questions: What do we want to learn from this cycle?	Can we get 100% of our students engaged in thinking, writing, sharing (pair or to class), and listening to, restating, and building on one another's ideas? Can they do it before any lessons on the topic? Does it help launch the topic?
Data: What information will we collecxt to answer our questions and test our prediction?	Students' responses both on their paper and shared out to the class poster. Seating chart tally as a record of who in each team is writing, pair sharing, sharing to class, and so on.
Results and Next Steps: What were the results? What did we learn? What will we do next?	This attempt was more successful than last time. I was able to use this to introduce a chapter as we first started looking at exponential functions. Every student wrote at least a couple on their page before sharing with groups/whole class, and each team shared out at least one idea. After this activity, they did the CPM leasson of exploring the exponential functions for different *b* values, and at the end of class we came we came back to this WODB slide and they said what new things they understood: for instance, what the equations for these four graphs could have been. I want to continue to find ways to tie this activity into the specific lesson they're about to do, as a landmark to visit before and after the lesson.

During his second PDSA cycle, Figure 7.2, he introduced the Which One Doesn't Belong activity as part of a warm-up in a different class period. Informed by the data in his first iteration, he modified his instruction. He incorporated visuals to help students "see" the relationship between multiplication and division in fractions. He found that his students were more engaged and that the use of visuals helped them think about the problem then articulate their reasoning. Through these cycles, he gained valuable knowledge (and evidence) that incorporating visuals into his lessons could engage the students and assist their learning. He indicated that he would continue to incorporate them into problem-solving activities, thus potentially improving his instructional practices. Depending on the degree to which these learnings changed his instructional norms, this instance of single-loop learning could also incite double-loop learning.

In addition to generating single-loop learnings through PDSA cycles, teachers also shared effective practices and resources with each other during network meetings, which could lead to improved instructional practices, as well. In one example during the April convening, teachers from multiple schools were engaging in inquiry and dialogue around their PDSA cycles. While one teacher shared a web-based graphing tool she used with her students, I observed two other teachers, who were from different schools, immediately navigate to the website on their laptops and ask her questions about how she applied the tool in the classroom. Building on this excitement and eagerness to learn new ideas from other schools, we structured our last convening as a showcase whereby selected teachers demonstrated the different resources they used during their PDSA cycles. Again, it was apparent during observations that teachers were enthused and engaged. The room was buzzing with on-task conversation and questions. One teacher shared in the survey, "I enjoyed today's session more than the previous one because there was a lot of designated time available to learn about different practices in greater detail and ask questions."

Learnings That Were Characteristic of Double-Loop Learning

While I cannot be sure that instructional theories-of-use were changing, there was evidence that teachers were reconsidering *how* they teach, versus merely looking for ways to improve their current practices of teaching. Their own PDSA forms, words, and behaviors provided the best indication of these shifting values, norms, strategies, and assumptions around student learning. According to Argyris and Schön (1996), it is this questioning of underlying values, norms, or strategies that will ultimately lead to more transformational change in practices.

Double-loop learning, or learnings with characteristics of double-loop learning, seemed to occur through the combination of math professional development and engaging in disciplined inquiry via the PDSA cycles. These experiences likely contributed to shifts in underlying instructional values and norms when it occurred.

FIGURE 7.2 ● Second PDSA Iteration for Sawyer Teacher, From February 6, 2018

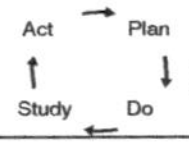

Act → Plan
↑ ↓ PDSA CYCLE FORM
Study ← Do

Change Idea	Describe: Which One Doesn't Belong What is the change: BStudents will "see" the realtionship between fraction division and multiplication. I will do a second WODB with the class, modifying the first WODB with more visual examples of fractions.
Predictions: What improvement do we think will happen?	Student will be more engaged, with students who do not normally get engaged with the activity. Students will understand the relationship between fractions and whole parts.
Questions: What do we want to learn from this cycle?	What are my students thinking about fractions, what concepts are easily seen, and which others are not?
Data: What information will we collect to answer our questions and test our prediction?	I will record the responses on the board. Students will create their own for homework.
Results and Next Steps: What were the results? What did we learn? What will we do next?	Student engagement was more apparent during this version of the activity. The drawings and figures were able to get more of the students enagaged and thinking about the problems. They were able to also find more creative answers and explain their reasoning better. I will use this info to help incorporate drawing into problem solving. Moving forward, I will now implement mixed numbers and operations through the use of the visual drawings.

In Tom's professional development sessions, he explained the philosophy behind the number sense routines and how to build on student learning. He had teachers assume the role of students during these activities to give them the perspective of how their students learned. During PDSA cycles, teachers posited certain predictions and reflected on evidence that confirmed or disconfirmed these notions. They tried multiple iterations of an idea and were presented with data on how new strategies and/or practices were more beneficial to student learning. They reconsidered certain practices and why they do them. Even in cases when teachers did not complete a PDSA cycle but still engaged in inquiry and dialogue with their colleagues, it spurred their own reflection about teaching practices.

The previous example in Figure 7.2 illustrated how double-loop learning could emerge from multiple PDSA iterations. A teacher from Roosevelt provided another example. He conducted four PDSA iterations around the general idea of group closure activities; those tasks that end a lesson. These activities can have multiple purposes, such as gauging student understanding and summarizing major points of a lesson. He conducted the four PDSA cycles over the course of approximately 6 to 7 weeks.

A review of his PDSA forms (not shown) showed how his thinking evolved through the process. For the first PDSA, he employed a team exit slip to assess student understanding. On reflection, he felt that the exit slip was easy to grade and fostered student discussion. Next, he experimented with another group closure activity where student groups wrote a summary of the day's lesson. He felt this activity also cultivated student discussion but expressed concern that his students did not exhibit a solid mathematical vocabulary in their written summaries. He decided to provide sentence starters for the written summaries in his next PDSA round. He found that, again, his students had a good discussion, but they demonstrated little academic mathematical language. From here, he wrote in his PDSA form that he planned to add a list of vocabulary words with the sentence starters for the fourth PDSA round. But then something changed. Instead of administering another iteration of the written summary group closure activity, he pivoted away from his initial idea and instead, had the students write their own problems. In his PDSA form, he described the process that led to his realization:

> *I really wanted to know what students were thinking and how they were problem solving. The group exit slip did not provide that information for each student. The group summaries were too general and it didn't provide me any information about their understanding or how they were thinking. So I thought having them create their own problem would give me better insight on their thinking and understanding.*

This teacher realized that exit tickets and written summaries did not provide him with enough information about student understanding. Somewhere along the process, there appeared to be a shift from wanting to know *what* his students knew, to *how* they think—a potential change in instructional values. My analysis cannot attribute this change to any particular event but it does represent a possible shift that was in line with Tom's vision of eliciting, understanding, and building on students' thinking.

Reconsidering instructional practices and underlying norms and values was particularly significant for teachers who only completed one or two PDSA cycles. These teachers seemed more reluctant to complete PDSA cycles and slower to embrace Tom's instructional vision, which was likely related to their teaching philosophies. Interviews with these teachers indicated that they tended to be more teacher-centered in their teaching styles rather than being student-centered. As previously discussed, they were also more likely to express concern regarding discipline and classroom management and may not have initially valued classroom experimentation as much as teachers who completed more PDSA cycles. Thus, these were the very teachers who needed to reconsider their assumptions about how students learn and why they taught the way they did.

In one example, a teacher who had not yet demonstrated a change in practices, and was hesitant to try a change idea in her classroom, was beginning to voice a new sentiment regarding student-centered learning. She often referred to herself as a "traditional teacher" and began the year expressing uncertainty about the school's more collaborative curriculum. Toward the end of the year, she articulated how network activities helped her see the value of student-to-student discussions:

> I mean, it [participating in the network] re-enforces what we're doing with this curriculum or the way the curriculum is set up. [It] is definitely a plus. Not just the content of math, but those soft skills about communication, and talking to each other, and putting that extra time.

In another case, a teacher who was very concerned about preventing his students from misbehaving and seemed reluctant to try a new idea in his classroom was beginning to show a greater inclination toward student-directed discussion. He explained:

> Well, I try to devote more time now to discussions, discussions amongst the students. We do these things, particularly with the warm-ups, and also when we're introducing a new concept. The idea of wait and think, think, pair, share. But just the idea of giving them a chance to talk about it and try if . . . Of course, if they really are talking about it. Then I just let it go for a while, and then, I use the "If you have one idea . . ." . . . Yeah, that's nice. The kids like it as something that they had not done before. But I mean, it's effective in that you can see what their ideas are and how many of them, you know, are thinking. I think just the idea of them again discussing the concept or the problem, how to apply the concept, it's taking a little more time with it. It's helpful.

While this teacher's quote signified a change in strategy within his usual instructional paradigm (warm-ups to existing lessons), it also indicates a deeper shift in values regarding his teaching style and learning about student thinking. His administrator confirmed the shift that he and other teachers were making in their instructional practices. Importantly, this was a school where Tom was also working with teachers through the Math Project. Teachers were getting more frequent exposure to Tom's instructional views. The administrator reported:

> *So they been doing grouping strategies, engagement strategies, much more mindfully and consistently this year than they had in the past. I don't know if they realize that's because they've been talking about it more and more exposed to it . . . I think he's just really mindful about incorporating those strategies into his instruction, as well. And then grouping stuff. So things that came out of the Math Project came out of [the network], he's definitely implementing. They're doing it, as well.*

Some teachers also demonstrated less student-deficit thinking and language. This indicated that these teachers were changing their mindsets, or at the very least questioning their underlying instructional values and norms. Several teachers began exhibiting more asset-based language during meetings. Others, who were initially very vocal in meetings about their students' lack of skills and knowledge, were now silent on the subject, suggesting that the group norm had shifted as well. Through his work with the teachers, including settings outside of the network, Tom was particularly cognizant of the language shifts:

> *That they might, might have been using more deficit language in the past, but now they're kind of thinking about like "Okay, so I have a lot within my locus of control that can actually influence how the kids engage with math." Um, I think implicitly they're understanding that, and it's kind of shifting their thinking about the kids as "They just don't know it, or they just disengage," to "Okay, there is something that they, they do know." What the very least, that now they're learning to not be so blatant about, like, their bias against kids. It's shifting in that sense, too. I'm hearing less language of, you know, "These kids just don't do this or don't do that." Which again, even that in itself is something that they're learning.*

The Importance of Reflective Structures for Single- and Double-Loop Learning

While the two previous sections illustrate single-loop learning and potential double-loop learning, and identify processes by which they occur (e.g., professional development, PDSA cycles), a more thorough discussion about reflection on practice is warranted as a potential mechanism of these learnings. Through network activities, teachers engaged in internal and external reflection that resulted in individual and team learnings, and teachers commonly attributed their learnings to this reflection time.

PDSA cycles offered a structure for experiential learning (Langley et al., 2009; Merriam & Bierema, 2014). More specifically, the converging of math instructional professional development with this PDSA format represented a reflective practice model of experiential learning. The reflective practice learning theory advances that learning occurs by reflecting on or in our practical experiences (Merriam & Bierema, 2014). More than 30 years ago, Schön (1983) posited that many professionals, including teachers, were faced with complex issues—the real-world of practice was messy—and that learning in practice was necessary to be successful (Merriam & Bierema, 2014). He believed that professional training alone was not enough to deal with this real-world complexity.

In our case, the PDSA cycle provided a format for trying new ideas, individual reflection, and dialogue and inquiry among colleagues. Teachers had a change idea, predicted the results, experimented in their classrooms, collected evidence, and compared their prediction with the actual results. Combining this format with Tom's number sense routines (or other change ideas) provided worthwhile content for them to put into practice and then reflect on. Learning commonly occurred through teachers' reflection on their experiences experimenting in their classroom, which is referred to as *reflection-on-action* in this model of experiential learning (Merriam & Bierema, 2014; Schön, 1983).

Learning through reflective practice can also occur by considering one's espoused theory against their theories-in-use, as previously discussed. The reflective structure of the PDSA also provided a vehicle for examining conflicts between espoused theory and theories-in-use, whether implicitly or explicitly, particularly through reflection on whether they met their prediction and why. This idea of confirming or disconfirming assumptions through the PDSA cycle is discussed more in the next section.

It was clear through teacher interviews, observations, and the end-of-year survey that the PDSA format facilitated both action and learning. One teacher, who was comfortable experimenting in her classroom before the network, acknowledged that this structure "reset" or reinvigorated her own practice. This sentiment was echoed by other teachers as well. This teacher explained:

> *I feel like, I've had a lot of priorities like, reset, um, I don't know how to say this. There are things in teaching that I like, have done, like, a couple of times, and I know that it works great, but then you just kind of don't do it because you're, like, trying to, you know, get through with all these other things. It's, you know, you're juggling a bunch of balls and whichever one gets closest to the ground is the one you're catching right now. But, you know, it was, it's been a nice opportunity to really have time to reflect and work on, "OK, what, what are the things I want to actually change, not just go along with how I've been doing it?" And that's been really fun.*

Other teachers expressed a similar appreciation for experimenting and reflecting in their practice through the survey. Teachers were asked an open-ended question, "Has participating in the network caused you to reflect on your own teaching practices? If so, how?" Almost half the teachers (7 out of 18) indicated that participating in the network caused them to see the value of trying or implementing new instructional practices, which was the most common answer given. Other answers acknowledged that teachers were thinking more about how to engage students and/or meet their students' needs (5 teachers). Specifically, one teacher expressed:

> *I have questioned why I do a lot of things in my practice to see if it is helping reach the end goal. I have reflected numerous times on the little changes that I make, or the new things I try (even if it's not my PDSA), to see how effective the practice is. I feel like I've tried more things in my practice than I did the last two years I've been at this school.*

As the network hub, we intentionally designed activities to foster meaningful questioning and reflection about their practices and PDSA cycles. We also aspired to aid learning for teachers who had not completed their own PDSA cycles. Specifically, we:

- provided opportunities for teachers to dialogue with colleagues within, and across, schools;

- explicitly taught productive inquiry and dialogue skills;

- strategically grouped teachers to foster dialogue and inquiry across schools, grouped teachers based on their personality and needs, and tried to combine teachers who we felt would connect and build relationships, provide valuable guidance, and/or who push each other's thinking;

- developed a productive inquiry and dialogue protocol to steer these conversations. This protocol included four timed steps:

  1. Teacher shared the results from their PDSA cycle.

  2. Other teachers asked clarifying questions and then more probing questions and/or suggestions to consider. Questions stems were provided.

  3. The initial teacher reflected on what they heard from the others.

  4. Once all teachers had their turn, they identified bright spots (what worked well) and additional questions for consideration.

Intentionally Designing Activities to Foster Double-Loop Learning

Although we did not intentionally design Tom's number sense routines to foster double-loop learnings, on our own reflection, we realized that these activities, combined with the PDSA format, promoted double-loop learning processes.

This was found in their advancing a prediction that they could confirm or disconfirm with evidence and coupling it with collective inquiry (Argyris & Schön, 1996). For example, during the initial causal analysis conducted in the fall, many teachers articulated deficit thinking regarding their students. They expressed opinions that many students were not interested in math, did not possess basic mathematical skills, could not do basic reasoning, and so on. Tom's Which One Doesn't Belong and choral counting routines challenged these deficit assumptions.

Through the PDSA process, some teachers predicted that they would see an increase in participation and engagement, and in some cases, 100% participation. What is important to note here is that many of the teachers making these predictions were the *same ones* who attributed students' lack of interest in math to the students. This suggested that their espoused theory (PDSA prediction) possibly conflicted with their actual theories-in-use (instruction that assumes these students were not participating because of their own lack of interest rather than the instructional practice, itself). Because the PDSA process required collecting observable evidence to assess whether they met their prediction, teachers in these examples collected data—students who participated in the activity, and what they said—and were often confronted with evidence that disconfirmed their initial theories-in-use. That is, the data suggested that more students were participating when the instructional activity engaged them in a different way. This was especially true when teachers iterated on the initial idea and provided opportunities for students to engage in multiple ways, such as writing individually or in a small group. As already discussed in this chapter, some teachers were shifting their own thinking, language, and instruction as result of these activities.

It is also important to note here that for a teacher to self- and group-reflect on this disconfirming evidence, it is extremely important that they are supported through either professional development and/or coaching, so they can successfully execute the activity. If a teacher cannot effectively implement the number sense routine, including knowing how to adjust when students need clarification or get stuck, they may be collecting evidence that confirms their student-deficit assumptions (i.e., attribute failure to their students, and not their own instructional gaps around the activity). Obviously, this would be detrimental to the learnings of the network.

Additionally, we recognized that PDSA inquiry and dialogue structures, whether within schools or network meetings, did not provide an abundance of time for teachers to engage in deeper discussions reflecting on the potential conflict between their espoused theories and theories-in-use. Each teacher typically had about 10 to 15 minutes to share their PDSA results and engage in inquiry and dialogue with their colleagues. Therefore, we decided that the network should promote these deeper discussions by intentionally creating the space and time.

At the April network convening, we designed an activity we called "circles of engagement." Teachers were grouped with teachers from other schools and asked to label some of their students by engagement level (not engaged, somewhat engaged, very engaged) and consider why they assigned those labels. Then they were asked to read a short article about middle school students' developmental needs and the classroom environment. University hub staff facilitated structured small group dialogue about the reading and teachers' own classroom experiences. Although, I have no evidence that this conversation resulted in double-loop learning, it spurred a lot of reflection and new dialogue around student experiences, and how teachers might better engage students. After the observation of two table discussions, it was clear these teachers were acknowledging that student engagement is a product of their own instructional practices. I heard teachers discuss how they could move students from the "not engaged" circle to the "very engaged circle" by using technology and giving students more varied opportunities to share their thinking and more ownership and choice in their learning. Teachers were engaging in authentic group dialogue, which was apparent by their ability to share their own views and acknowledge and question the perspectives of the article and other teachers.

Conclusion

The ultimate purpose of improvement networks is to generate collective learnings that can improve complex problems of practice. In education, these complex problems can be related to deficit-oriented instructional patterns, which may be tied to educators underlying values and norms. As such, improving persistent educational problems may require more than single-loop learning. All learning is not created equal. Network improvement communities should cultivate double-loop learning through PDSA cycles and thoughtful reflective and inquiry structures that provide opportunities for teachers to collect evidence that confirm or disconfirm their instructional assumptions.

Questions for Discussion

1. Why is double-loop learning important for fostering transformative change?

2. How does reflection foster double-loop learning?

3. In your own settings or organizations, what structures, if any, are in place to promote reflection?

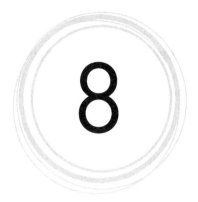

Lessons and Reflections From a Case Study

I embarked on this project with the goal of providing an improvement science road map for anyone aspiring to use these methods to effect positive change and as an example of evaluation in practice. However, through the process of researching and writing this book, I now have a deeper understanding of what it means to drive change in complex systems. This chapter summarizes the key lessons from the case study, grounded in empirical data, as well as lessons learned from current reflections on what we could have done differently. Furthermore, I connect the case study to the concepts introduced in Part 1 of this book to foster our understanding of how to lead change in complex systems.

In this chapter, I cover:

- Lessons From Theory, Research, and Practice: Findings From the Case Study

- Lessons From Continued Practice: Additional Reflections

- Bringing It All Together: Learning From Astronauts, Elephants, Einstein, and Teachers

- Moving Forward in a Complex World

Lessons From Research and Practice: Findings From the Case Study

Several important lessons for implementing improvement science initiatives were learned through the findings from the empirical case study and can be extrapolated to other organizations and settings outside of education.

Lesson 1: Build Capacity Through Merging

The initiative benefited from expertise in three disparate areas: improvement science (profound knowledge and evaluative inquiry methods), subject knowledge (math instruction), and knowledge of relationship dynamics within the schools. A team of complementing experts not only provides unique expertise in their respective areas, but also merges knowledge in a way that elevates the hub's ability to build capacity. The whole is greater than the sum of its parts.

Lesson 2: Combine Visions

Building on the first point, the synergistic nature of a team of experts working closely together helped the teachers learn improvement science. Tom had a vision of quality math instruction. I had a vision for building improvement science capacity. When our two visions intertwined, teachers were able to learn improvement science methods within the context of real-world math instruction, which is what they really wanted to learn. By framing the improvement science tools around the math instructional professional development, teachers were able to transfer their learning and construct meaning and make sense of improvement science concepts that might have otherwise seemed disconnected and abstract (Brown et al., 1989; Merriam & Bierema, 2014; Preskill & Boyle, 2008).

Lesson 3: Meetings Matter

Assuming administrators and teachers will make time to meet or utilize existing collaboration time may be unrealistic given their competing priorities. In schools where administrators were not fully involved, it was more difficult to schedule regular meetings and the case study found that the number of completed Plan, Do, Study, Act (PDSA) cycles per school was directly related to the number of times the hub met with teachers at their schools. Supportive administrators' cooperation and assistance is key to teachers' ability to implement improvement science activities.

Lesson 4: Foster and Facilitate Authentic and Productive Conversations

One should not assume that merely establishing regular meetings is enough. Teachers who indicated they already met regularly during department meetings or common conference periods did not frequently discuss student learning or solicit feedback from their peers regarding their own teaching practices. They may have restrictive or loose meeting structures that deter or even discourage inquiry with one another. Furthermore, teachers may not have the capacity or comfort level to teach and facilitate improvement science activities to each other. An outside facilitator can encourage open conversations and help them feel supported in peer-to-peer inquiry.

Lesson 5: Foster Double-Loop Learning Through PDSA Cycles

The PDSA format sparks a reflective practice mechanism that contributes to both single-loop and double-loop learnings, but it is the double-loop learning aspect that is especially powerful. In the case of this network, combining the reflective structure of the PDSA with an intentional instructional practice learned through professional development cultivated double-loop learning. The evidence suggested that teachers, who initially felt some students would "never" be interested in mathematics, were now reconsidering their own role in their students' engagement. The PDSA cycle provided evidence that these students were, in fact, engaging in the activity. This gave teachers cause to reflect on their underlying instructional theories-in-use.

Lesson 6: Building Improvement Science Capacity

Lessons 1 through 5 inform Lesson 6, which is the crux of the case study's research problem; that is, how can we build capacity for those closest the problem to engage in improvement work. As discussed earlier in the book, building this knowledge and skills in evaluative or improvement methods is one of the key challenges faced when engaging in participatory frameworks. Because Lesson 6 was the overarching case study objective, I devote more space to our discussion of what we learned through this lesson.

As discussed earlier in this book, the case study's conceptual framework was grounded in Preskill and Boyle's (2008) multidisciplinary capacity building model and Argyris and Schön's (1996) concepts of single-loop and double-loop learning. From the case study's empirical data and findings, Preskill and Boyle's model can be extended into the improvement science realm (Rohanna, in press). In this case, the model is specific to networks but can also be applied to other organizational endeavors. Figure 8.1 offers this new improvement science capacity building model, with the intent of providing guidance to others hoping to lead improvement science initiatives.

The focus in Year 1 should be on building improvement science capacity, shown in the first box. This goal is supported by identifying two visions: one regarding the subject knowledge, and one regarding the improvement science capacity. These visions are furthered by evaluation capacity building teaching and learning strategies (Preskill & Boyle, 2008), shown at the bottom of the model, and experiential learning theories, shown at the top of the model. Situated cognition learning theory (learning in context), as a learning mechanism, contributes to both organizational and individual capacity development (Box 2). The learning transpires through subject matter professional development, improvement science professional development, and in-school meetings facilitated by an improvement science specialist.

Once the network starts building improvement science capacity, it will generate learnings, which are conceptualized as single-loop and double-loop learnings (Box 3). These learnings are generated through professional development,

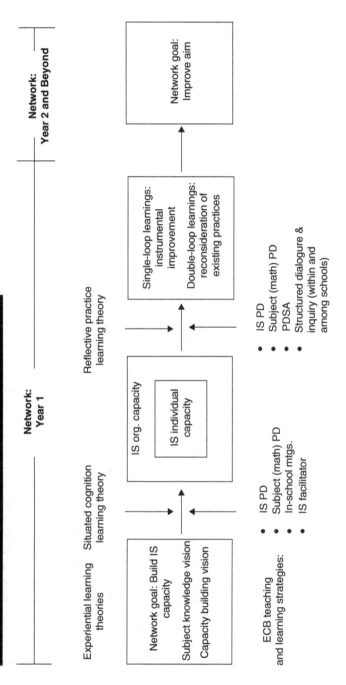

FIGURE 8.1 ● Improvement Science Capacity Building Model

PDSA cycles, and structured inquiry and dialogue among teachers. Structured reflective practice is the underlying learning mechanism that drives the single-loop and double-loop learnings.

The model further posits that these intermediate outcomes—building improvement science capacity and generating learnings—need to occur before improving the network aim or problem of practice. The focus in Year 2 and beyond can shift to improving the aim. Since this model is based on empirical data from Year 1, the box under Year 2 has not been further populated.

It should be noted that the findings from this case study, and thus this model, suggest one viable explanation with the presence of equifinality. That is, there could be other factors and mechanisms, or combinations of these, that could lead to the same outcomes. This book only claims these findings as one potential path to derive these outcomes.

Lessons From Continued Practice: Additional Reflections

Change does not roll in on the wheels of inevitability,
but comes through continuous struggle.

—Martin Luther King, Jr.

Three years later, the network still exists. While we shifted our focus to improving our aim in Year 2, outcomes are mixed. Grades data for the first 2 years of the network showed that many teachers made progress toward their aim of increasing the percentage of students passing with a C grade or better, while others did not.[1] However, changes in outcomes take time, and we are encouraged by the changes we see in teacher mindset and practices.

Our team remains responsive to new challenges and insights that emerge every day. Transformational change in complex systems requires a reconsideration of values and practices by its actors. We regularly reflect on our lessons learned and what we can do differently. To that point, I offer three additional lessons learned; what I wish I knew in that first year that I know now.

Lesson 7: Also Focus on School Team Culture

While we did work with teams individually at their schools—and through this process we created structures and fostered more productive collaboration—we could have focused more on building individual school team culture in addition to the network's culture. For some teams, trust came naturally through the collaborative structures we oversaw, but for others it did not. Stronger school teams sat together at network meetings, while other teams broke into smaller groups or pairs and sat apart. The siloed teams did

---

[1]Due to COVID-19, data on grades for the end of Year 3 were not available.

not tend to collaborate with each other unless we provided structures that placed them together.

Working with school teams today, we facilitate the development of community agreements immediately to further teambuilding and a collaborative culture. Community agreements, as defined by the National Equity Project (n.d.), are

> a consensus on what every person in our group needs from each other and commits to each other in order to feel safe, supported, open, productive and trusting . . . so that we can serve our students (or clients) well, do our best work, and achieve our common vision . . .

These are different than norms. Norms often seek to establish rules that govern behavior at meetings or group functions. Community agreements seek to establish a more relational aspect, and for members to be open about their needs to feel comfortable engaging in authentic dialogue with each other.

We also establish core team beliefs and values. In our work in education, we ask administrators and teachers to first reflect on their own identities to help them understand how they see themselves as individuals, before developing a team identity. Then we ask them to share their core beliefs around teaching and learning. We facilitate a process to build team core values through dialogue and activities. These conversations also serve to identify underlying assumptions or values that administrators and teachers may hold around student learning.

These are small steps that can have a big impact. They foster trust. Individuals share their hopes and dreams, as well their own stories and challenges. These activities foster a sense that everyone is committed to positive change (e.g., helping students), even if they disagree on how to achieve it. In my own experience, I have seen people willing to speak up and push each other's thinking and engage in real dialogue if they feel this sense of trust and regard for each other. Stating core team beliefs and values upfront can also help teams reach consensus or make decisions. The team commits to only engaging in strategies or activities that are aligned with their core values.

Lesson 8: Analyze Each School's Complex System Patterns

In the case of the network, we bounded the system to each teacher's classroom. It was manageable and within their locus of control, thereby creating a sense of efficacy in their ability to make change. We also used the fishbone diagram as a tool for causal systems analysis to better understand why students were failing math classes, considering challenges across the system. We still do this today. We created the space for teachers to experiment through PDSA cycles. We also still do this today. However, one aspect that was missing in our network was a deeper consideration of system patterns that exist within complex social systems and how they can hinder change.

Schools exist in complex systems. We cannot predict cause and effect relationships, or how change will happen, because administrators and teachers are semi-independent. They can be influenced but not controlled (nor should they).

Diagramming causal feedback loops, whether reinforcing or balancing, provides an invaluable understanding why change may not occur in schools despite our best efforts (Senge, 2006; Stroh, 2015). Each school (or organization) may have a different system pattern, or they may all have a common one. For example, in Chapter 2, I provided the example of a district getting stuck in the status quo because they were continually responding to a target assessment score but not accepting the time it took to change. They got stuck in "adopt, attack, abandon," a common pattern in schools today.

Complex systems are characterized by unpredictability, but there are patterns. As a network, we bounded the problem and the system within teachers' locus of control, but it was also crucial to understand other system patterns and create a space for all stakeholders to diagnose and discuss those patterns together. In the case of the network, analyzing system patterns at the administrator level may have helped school leaders better understand their role rather than primarily relying on teachers to change their practices in the classroom.

For those leading change initiatives, analyzing underlying system patterns furthers understanding about where change can get *stuck*. For example, if teachers are aiming at an assessment target (e.g., 90% of students achieve at grade level) and not achieving it, they may get stuck in the status quo via a "Fixes that Fail" or "Shifting the Burden" system archetype. Understanding these patterns provides more understanding for how to get *unstuck*.

Lesson 9: Champion Innovative, Equitable Measures

The above is an example of a system potentially reorienting itself *away* from transformational change using traditional data: data focused on improving the percentage of students performing at grade level. While understandable, this focus keeps attention on students (shifting the burden) rather than instructional practices and policies. Often traditional measures accepted by those in power or leadership, whether for accountability or performance monitoring, are also most accessible or practical. Transformational systems change may require taking a risk on data and measures not traditionally viewed as established, objective, or *hard*.

In their book, *The Dance of Change: A Fifth Discipline Fieldbook for Mastering the Challenges of Learning Organizations,* Senge and colleagues (1999) discuss measurement and assessment as a limiting process for innovative changes, potentially resulting in a "limits to growth" system pattern: "How do people judge whether something new is working? . . . In fact, significant new business practices may contradict the thinking behind many traditional measures" (p. 281–282). Further, they explain that those asserting the need for new measures, instead of established traditional measures, may be seen as trying to avoid accountability.

In the case of the network, we faced this contradiction. We were trying to transform classroom practices, ideally leading to more equitable practices (implicit in meeting the needs of all students) but we faced challenges identifying meaningful measures that were common across all schools. Grades were established as a measurement. However, grades are often systemically inequitable. We encouraged teachers to focus on changing the drivers but because grades were on the driver diagram, they remained a focal area.

The use of grades, which are often subjective and can perpetuate systemic inequities, was more than a measurement problem. In fact, as we discussed the use of grades for our aim in Year 1 in the context of reliability, we decided that although not ideal, using grades was acceptable providing that each school and teacher only compared the change over time to themselves. We assumed teachers would be somewhat consistent in how they graded, year-to-year. What we did not fully discuss, however, was the idea that grades could be inequitable in addition to being inconsistent, thereby contradicting what we hoped to improve. And by focusing on grades as the ultimate aim, we were essentially limiting our growth in developing equitable instructional practices, an implicit goal in Years 1 and 2 of the network that we made more explicit in Year 3.

Therefore, in Year 4, we made changes to our aim and how we collect data. The new aim explicitly shifts the focus from grades to the use of equitable instructional practices. The challenge is how to measure, and measure consistently, across multiple schools. We decided that the university hub team would conduct classroom observations using a structured tool designed to gather data on equitable instructional practices in math that aligned with the primary drivers.

After three challenging years of trying to find or create practical measures that teachers can readily gather, we decided that the hub needed to own this responsibility. Data regarding equitable practices does not exist and is not easy to collect. It is not a traditional measure. But it is crucial for transforming our system. To obtain one common measure for the network, thereby also allowing us to set a network target and make the Year 4 process feasible for the hub team, we plan to sample classrooms across the schools rather than observe them all.

Bringing It All Together: Learning From Astronauts, Elephants, Einstein, and Teachers

In the case study, we saw how improving persistent problems in complex systems requires disciplined, formative, and continuous inquiry that is responsive to arising challenges. Successfully engaging in this inquiry requires dedicated time and structures that promote authentic dialogue and productive collaboration. We also learned that context is never static in complex systems: What works in one part of the system might not work in another, and what works at one point in time might not work at another. Complexity science suggests that solutions need to emerge through continuous real-world experiments conducted in a safe space where failure is an opportunity to learn. Because actors are always adapting, and very little can be predicted, emergence is the name of the game. In the case of the network, improvement science provided the tools and structures to learn and respond to that emergence. Teachers were encouraged to use PDSA cycles to experiment with different instructional strategies in their classrooms. The PDSA cycle helped them generate new knowledge and iterate to fit the practice to their own context, and importantly, helped them reconsider their underlying assumptions around how students learn. As in the example of the Apollo 13 lunar module controllers, teachers had the safe space to learn and experiment, allowing them to learn and reflect on each new challenge that arose in their classrooms.

We also affirmed that leading change in complex systems requires an inclusive participatory approach. The case study illustrates how the network merged improvement, subject, and specific school knowledge and embraced the experiences of those closest to the problem (i.e., the teachers). Systems thinking necessitates the perspectives, knowledge, and experiences of many in the system. As with the blind men and the elephant, limited perspectives will lead to an erroneous understanding of the whole system. The elephant is not only "like a wall," or "like a rope." Only by putting all perspective together can we see the whole.

Albert Einstein once said, "We cannot solve our problems with the same thinking we used when we created them." This rang true that day in the library, when teachers were brainstorming ideas for teaching students a "lacking skill" by using their existing instructional paradigm. They did not know another way to approach the problem, but Tom, an expert and outsider, did. His guidance supported them to try new practices that engaged students in different ways, and thus, fostered the double-loop learning necessary for transformational change. Tom's expertise and vision of quality mathematics instruction was responsible for breaking up *same thinking* and showed that the inclusive participatory approach can benefit when it includes those outside the system.

It would be a mistake, however, to *only* listen to those outside the system. In our case, we met regularly with teachers to understand the problem from their perspective. We co-created our driver diagram by merging research with areas they identified for growth and improvement. We continually learned from them how to best support their own goals (e.g., move more quickly from the understanding the problem phase to taking action and experimenting with strategies). And importantly, they helped us learn what wasn't working (e.g., the data collection rubric).

Another case in point: Newark Public Schools. The voices of crucial system actors (e.g., parents, teachers, principals) were dismissed by *mostly* well-meaning outsiders intent on grabbing "the system by the roots," "yanking it out," and starting over (Russakoff, 2014, p. 58). Imagine how that story might have ended if parents, teachers, and principals were consulted to understand the problems before the outsiders jumped to inaccurate conclusions and ill-conceived solutions. And imagine if teachers and principals had been given the opportunity to learn, experiment, and reflect on potential strategies under the guidance of improvement and content experts, like in this book's case study. The example of the Newark Public Schools is a cautionary tale we all should heed when leading change.

Moving Forward in a Complex World

Well, where do we go from here? If you've made it to the end of this book, I assume you're someone who hopes to make positive change in this world and, like many of us, struggles with how to improve a persistent problem in a complex system. This book shared both theory and practice in hopes of supporting you, whether you're an evaluator, practitioner, or graduate student. My hope is that this book gave you an opportunity to reflect more deeply on formative evaluative methods—particularly continuous improvement endeavors grounded in improvement science—and how they can be applied to your own contexts.

Moving forward in a complex world requires continuous inquiry and learning. Leading change in complex systems of our creation is difficult but also not impossible. Like Ernő Rubik who invented a puzzle that even he could not immediately solve, it requires an understanding of the puzzle pieces: system dynamics, continuous participatory approaches, and informed methods for improvement. These are evaluative concepts that can be leveraged for social change. By understanding these pieces, we are well positioned to lead this charge and solve society's most puzzling problems.

Questions for Discussion

1. Consider the lessons learned in this chapter. Which one of these, if any, most resonates with your own experiences?

2. Why do you think the model promotes the need to focus on capacity-building for the first year rather than improving outcomes?

3. Albert Einstein once said, "We cannot solve our problems with the same thinking we used when we created them." Why is this an important consideration when leading change?

• Appendix •
Case Study Methodology

Setting

The University served as the hub for the network. The network was housed in the University's School of Education. The University team included the associate dean as the project director, a math coach, an improvement science specialist (me), and two school liaisons. My role was elevated to network coordinator mid-year when I took a larger role in the planning and presentation of network content. The initial focus of the network was to improve student outcomes in Algebra I and was later expanded to include all middle school math. The University began planning the network in the fall of 2016, and it was launched at the beginning of the 2017–2018 school year. Seven network convenings were held throughout Year 1.

Five schools were recruited to participate in the network in the spring of 2017. These schools resided in one large urban school district in Southern California. There was one K–12 school, one high school, two middle schools (sixth grade to eighth grade), and one junior high (sixth grade to ninth grade). Within these schools, math teachers from each of the relevant grades participated in the network. Administrators were also invited and participated to varying degrees.

Case Study Design

This study employed an explanatory, single case study approach with embedded school units (Yin, 2014). A case study was most appropriate for this study because its purpose was to examine the phenomenon of how to prepare schools to successfully participate in a networked improvement community within the real-life context of which it occurred (Yin, 2014). The primary outcome of a success was specified as the completion of Plan, Do, Study, Act (PDSA) cycles by schools, with individual teachers completing their own PDSA cycles. The networked improvement community, as the single case, was bounded by the activities occurring through the end of the network's first year. The embedded school units were also bounded by only including the people and activities related to the network.

A single case study, and more specifically this particular network case, was deemed appropriate for two reasons. First, because of my positioning as both a researcher and a graduate student researcher (GSR) supporting the network, I had intimate access to the decision making, planning, and processes of this particular network. This access provided the opportunity for a detailed examination of how to prepare schools to successfully participate in the network, including how to build improvement science capacity, which had not been undertaken before in an empirical study of networked improvement communities. Second, the network represented a common case. The network hub was a research institution, whose network was grant-funded, that recruited public schools to participate. Thus, it was foreseeable that this network was a usual case and provided an opportunity to capture the conditions and circumstances of a typical network situation.

This case study is further specified as a single case study with embedded school units (Yin, 2014), because this, and any networked improvement community in education, consists of distinct schools. Because the research sought to explain how schools can be prepared to successfully participate in a networked improvement community, this study's analysis occurs at multiple levels (i.e., the completion of PDSA cycles by individual schools and by the network as a whole). This design required data collected from hub staff, network convenings, school meetings, and teachers and administrators, along with network and school artifacts.

Participant Selection and Recruitment

By the end of Year 1, the network hub team consisted of five people. Three of these individuals—the project director, the math coach, and the school liaison—were recruited into the study because they represented the core team members who were present throughout the year. (I represented the improvement science specialist.) These individuals were recruited for interviews via email and in-person conversations.

All five schools were included in the case study to obtain more potential outcome variation (# of PDSA cycles completed by school), as well as obtaining a wider range of capacities, structures, and conditions that could explain outcome variations. The general characteristics of the five network schools are shown in Table A1.1. The grade level ranges for each school are not shown due to the increased likelihood of identifying schools based on this characteristic.

The interviews further employed purposive sampling. Eight teachers and administrators from three schools—Middleview, Sawyer, and Central—were interviewed as part of this study. These schools were selected because they included teachers within a school that had the most variation in the number of PDSA cycles completed by mid-April of Year 1. The purpose of this sampling technique was to gather data related to school and individual capacity differences. Two teachers from each school were recruited via email. Of those, one teacher from each school represented either an individual who completed a "high" number of PDSA cycles or a "low" number.

School	Number of network teachers	Total students	Demographics (%)					
			Low SES	Afr. Am.	Asian	Hisp./ Lat.	White	Other
Roosevelt	6	1,004	91.8	1.7	9.7	80.8	1.6	6.2
Marshall	6	613	56.3	20.6	5.2	40.6	28.1	5.5
Middleview	4	394	77.9	51.5	0	46.7	0.3	1.5
Sawyer	4	660	75.3	13.0	3.5	69.2	10.9	3.4
Central	3	1,564	75.6	24.6	7.0	52.9	11.6	3.9

TABLE A1.1 ● Network School Characteristics, 2017–2018

Note: Source is the California Department of Education. The number of teachers represents those participating in the network in May 2018.

Data Collection

This multiple-method case study examined and triangulated data from surveys, interviews, observations, and documents and/or artifacts. Due to my own positionality and the potential bias that could ensue, it was important to include a variety of data and methods to increase the credibility of my findings (Guba & Lincoln, 1986). Because this case study developed a process-tracing narrative (George & Bennett, 2005), it was also vital to collect an abundance of data from multiple sources to generate this detailed narrative. Furthermore, as Yin (2014) points out, incorporating multiple methods into case studies allows the researcher to collect a stronger array of evidence than could be obtained by any single method alone, thus, further strengthening the findings against my own potential biases. Table A1.2 first shows the data sources, with each category further described in this section.

Analysis

The analysis followed a multistep process. Data sources were first analyzed individually using the relevant techniques. For example, interviews were coded using a structural coding scheme for the first-cycle codes (Saldaña, 2013). The process not only used a priori codes from the conceptual framework and research questions, but also allowed for more inductive descriptive, versus, and process coding in an additional round of first-cycle coding. Pattern coding was used for the second-cycle coding, with some cases retaining their initial structural code, and other cases acquiring a new pattern code developed by

TABLE A1.2 ● Data Sources for Case Study
Network Sources
• Interviews: network hub team (3 interviews)
• Observations of network convenings (6 observations)
• Surveys (2)
• Documents/Artifacts
• Convening agenda, presentation materials, feedback forms
• Causal analyses artifacts: fishbone diagram, process maps
• Worksheets from meeting activities
• Network driver diagram
• GSR notes and calendar
School Sources
• Interviews: Teachers and administrators (9 interviews)
• Participant observations of school network-related meetings (23 observations)
• Documents/Artifacts
• Fishbone diagrams, process maps, beginning driver diagrams
• PDSA forms
• Secondary data: demographic, enrollment, and achievement data from the California Dept. of Education

Note: Three of the network convening observations were conducted by someone other than myself due to my role leading those meetings. GSR notes and calendar are my own.

combining lower level codes into higher level categories. Observations were also coded using a similar deductive/inductive approach. Surveys were descriptively analyzed due to their small sample sizes (n = 23, n = 19). Each PDSA cycle was systematically analyzed in Excel to determine if the change idea was aligned to the network's theory of change (driver diagram), and whether the completed PDSA was indicative of single-loop or double-loop learning. The documents, artifacts, and demographic data were also analyzed and incorporated to provide additional context for the case. One researcher conducted all coding and analysis.

The case study utilized detailed narrative process tracing methods to answer the research questions. Process tracing is a within-case analytical technique for identifying causal mechanisms that lead to an outcome for a single case (George & Bennett, 2005). Process tracing techniques are commonly used in political science for their ability to study the causes of a single event or case, while recognizing there could be alternative causal paths to the same outcome (George & Bennett, 2005). The analysis also utilized within-case, cross-unit (schools) analysis that generated additional evidence related to variation in

PDSA cycle completion by schools and teachers. Last, to further strengthen the validity of the study, additional tests of empirical data were conducted on the findings by systematically considering a wide range of alternative explanations and what evidence would be expected if the findings were true (or not true).

Limitations

This case study, like other research studies, has a few notable limitations. One limitation of this study is that it is a single case study that was selected by convenience (i.e., the University network). To address this potential generalizability limitation, I employed a nested case study design by embedding the schools and conducted cross-school analyses to identify and explain variations within the one network case. Additionally, I incorporated theory to help explain the mechanisms that led to the successful outcome of the network (i.e., situated cognition and reflective practice experiential learning theories). According to Yin (2014) and George and Bennett (2005), the use of these theories strengthens the ability to make generalizations from one case.

This study is also limited because it represents one cluster of schools, within a Southern California metropolitan area. These schools may not reflect the experiences of schools from other parts of the country. Furthermore, this network was an instructionally based networked improvement community focused on building the improvement science capacity of teachers and schools. This specific focus could limit the model's generalizability to other types of networked improvement communities that are less intent on building teacher capacity.

• References •

Alkin, M. C. (1991). Evaluation theory development: II. In M. W. McLaughlin & D. C. Phillips (Eds.), *Evaluation and education: At quarter century* (Ninetieth yearbook of the National Society for the Study of Education, pp. 91–112). University of Chicago Press.

Alkin, M. C., & Vo, A. T. (2018). *Evaluation essentials from A to Z* (2nd ed.). Guilford Press.

American Evaluation Association Systems in Evaluation Topical Interest Group. (2018). *Principals for effective use of systems thinking in evaluation.* https://www.systemsinevaluation.com/welcome/setig-principles-document-now-available/

American Society for Quality. (2020a). *The define, measure, analyze, improve, control (DMAIC) process.* https://asq.org/quality-resources/dmaic

American Society for Quality. (2020b). *What is lean?* https://asq.org/quality-resources/dmaic

Argyris, C., & Schön, D. A. (1996). *Organizational learning II: Theory, method and practice.* Addison-Wesley.

Berwick, D. M. (2008). The science of improvement. *Journal of the American Medical Association, 299*(10), 1182–1184.

Brown, J. S., Collins, A., & Duguid, P. (1989). Situated cognition and the culture of learning. *Educational Researcher, 18*(1), 32–42.

Bryk, A. S. (2009). Support a science of improvement. *Phi Delta Kappan, 90*(8), 597–600.

Bryk, A. S., Gomez, L. M., Grunow, A., & LeMahieu, P. G. (2015). *Learning to improve: How America's schools can get better at getting better.* Harvard Education Press.

California Community Colleges Chancellor's Office (2020a). Home. https://www.cccco.edu/

California Community Colleges Chancellor's Office (2020b). Vision for success. https://www.cccco.edu/About-Us/Vision-for-Success

California Department of Education. (2017a). California assessment of student performance and progress: Smarter balanced assessment [Data file]. https://caaspp.cde.ca.gov/sb2017/Search

California Department of Education. (2017b). K–12 Public school enrollment time series [Data file]. https://dq.cde.ca.gov/dataquest/

Carpenter, T. P., Fennema, E., Franke, M. L., Levi, L., & Empson, S. B. (1999). *Children's mathematics: Cognitively guided instruction.* Heinemann.

Cass, S. (2005). *Apollo 13, we have a solution* (Parts 1, 2, and 3). https://spectrum.ieee .org/tech-history/space-age/apollo-13-we-have-a-solution   https://spectrum.ieee .org/tech-history/space-age/apollo-13-we-have-a-solution-part-2   https://spectrum .ieee.org/tech-history/space-age/apollo-13-we-have-a-solution-part-3

Centers for Disease Control and Prevention. (2020a, March 19). Overdose death rates involving opioids, by type, United States 2000–2017. https://www.cdc.gov/ drugoverdose/data/analysis.html

Centers for Disease Control and Prevention (2020b, March 19). Three waves of opioid overdose deaths. https://www.cdc.gov/drugoverdose/epidemic/index .html#three-waves

Christie, C. A., Inkelas, M., & Lemire, S. (Eds.). (2017, Spring). *Improvement science in evaluation: Methods and uses* (New directions for evaluation, vol. 153). John Wiley & Sons.

Clyburn, G. M. (2013). Improving on the American dream: Mathematics pathways to student success. *Change: The Magazine of Higher Learning, 45*(5), 15–23.

Cousins, J. B. (2003). Utilization effects of participatory evaluation. In T. Kellaghan & D. L. Stufflebeam (Eds.), *International handbook of educational evaluation* (pp. 245–266). Kluwer Academic Publishers.

Cousins, J. B., & Earl, L. M. (1992). The case for participatory evaluation. *Educational Evaluation and Policy Analysis, 14*(4), 397–418.

Cronbach, L. (1963). Course improvement through evaluation. *Teachers College Record, 64*, 672–683. Reprinted in D. L. Stufflebeam, G. F. Madaus, & T. Kellaghan (Eds.). (2000). *Evaluation Models* (pp. 235–247). Kluwer.

Deming, W. E. (2018). *Out of the crisis.* MIT Press.

Deming, W. E. (1994). *The new economics* (2nd ed.). MIT Press.

Dewey, J. (1963). *Experience and education.* Macmillan.

Engelbart, D. C. (1992). Toward high-performance organizations: A strategic role for groupware. *Proceedings of GroupWare '92 Conference.* Morgan Kaufmann.

George, A. L., & Bennett, A. (2005). *Case studies and theory development in the social sciences.* MIT Press.

Guba, E. G., & Lincoln, Y. S. (1986). But is it rigorous? Trustworthiness and authenticity in naturalistic evaluation. *New Directions for Program Evaluation, 1986*(30), 73–84. doi:10.1002/ev.1427

The Health Foundation. (2011). *Report: Improvement science.* https://www.health.org .uk/publications/improvement-science

Hinnant-Crawford, B. N. (2020). *Improvement science in education: A primer.* Myers Education Press.

Huang, M. (January 2018). 2016–2017 Impact report: Six years of results from the Carnegie Math Pathways. Carnegie Foundation for the Advancement of Teaching. https://www.carnegiefoundation.org/resources/publications/2016-2017-impact-report-six-years-of-results-from-the-carnegie-math-pathways/

Kurtz, C. F., & Snowden D. J. (2003). The new dynamics of strategy: Sense-making in a complex and complicated world. *IBM Systems Journal, 42*(3), 462–483.

Kotlowitz, A. (2015, August 19). 'The prize,' by Dale Russakoff. *New York Times*. https://www.nytimes.com/2015/08/23/books/review/the-prize-by-dale-russakoff.html

Labin, S., Duffy, L., Meyers, D., Wandersman, A., & Lesesne, C. (2012). A research synthesis of the evaluation capacity building literature. *American Journal of Evaluation, 33*(3), 307–338.

Langley, G. J., Moen, R. D., Nolan, K. M., Nolan, T. W., Norman, C. L., & Provost, L. P. (2009). *The improvement guide: A practical approach to enhancing organizational performance* (2nd ed.). Jossey-Bass.

Lemire, S., Christie, C.A., & Inkelas, M. (2017). The methods and tools of improvement science. In C. A. Christie, M. Inkelas, & S. Lemire (Eds.), *Improvement science in evaluation: Methods and uses* (New directions for evaluation, vol. 153, pp. 23–33). Jossey-Bass and the American Evaluation Association.

The Lesson Study Group at Mills College. (2018). *About lesson study.* https://lesson-research.net/about-lesson-study/what-is-lesson-study/

Lockwood, M., Dillman, M., & Boudett, K. P. (2017). R&D: Using data wisely at the system level. *Phi Delta Kappan, 99*(1), 25–30. http://kappanonline.org/using-data-wisely-system-level/

Martin, L., Laderman, M., Hyatt, J., & Krueger J. (2016, April). *Addressing the opioid crisis in the United States*. IHI Innovation Report. Institute for Healthcare Improvement. http://www.ihi.org/resources/Pages/Publications/Addressing-Opioid-Crisis-US.aspx

Meadows, D. (2008). *Thinking in systems: A primer* (D. Wright, Ed.). Chelsea Green.

Mejia, M. C., Rodriguez, O., & Johnson, H. (2019, October). *What happens when colleges broaden access to transfer-level courses? Evidence from California's community colleges.* Public Policy Institute of California. https://www.ppic.org/wp-content/uploads/what-happens-when-colleges-broaden-access-to-transfer-level-courses-evidence-from-californias-community-colleges.pdf

Mejia, M. C., Rodriguez, O., & Johnson, H. (2016, November). *Preparing students for success in California's community colleges.* Public Policy Institute of California. https://www.ppic.org/content/pubs/report/R_1116MMR.pdf

Merriam, S. B., & Bierema, L. L. (2014). *Adult learning: Linking theory and practice.* Jossey-Bass.

Midgley, G. (2007). Systems thinking for evaluation. In B. Williams & I. Iman (Eds.), *Systems concepts in evaluation: An expert anthology* (pp. 11–34). EdgePress.

Moen, R. D., & Norman, C. L. (2010, November). Circling back: Clearing up myths about the Deming cycle and seeing how it keeps evolving. *Quality Progress, 22–28.* http://www.apiweb.org/circling-back.pdf

National Council of Teachers of Mathematics. (2014). *Principles to actions: Ensuring mathematical success for all.* Author.

National Equity Project. (n.d.). *Developing community agreements.* https://www .nationalequityproject.org/tools/developing-community-agreements

Park, S., Hironaka, S., Carver, P., & Nordstrum, L. (2013). *Continuous improvement in education.* Carnegie Foundation for the Advancement of Teaching. https://www .carnegiefoundation.org/wp-content/uploads/2014/09/carnegie-foundation_ continuous-improvement_2013.05.pdf

Parsons, B. (2012). *Using complexity science concepts when designing system interventions and evaluation.* InSites. http://insites.org/resource/using-complexity-science-concepts-when-designing-system-interventions-and-evaluations/

Patton, M.Q. (2011). *Developmental evaluation: Applying complexity concepts to enhance innovation and use.* Guilford Press.

Patton, M.Q. (1996). A world larger than formative and summative. *Evaluation Practice, 17*(2), 131–144.

Patton, M. Q. (1994). Developmental evaluation. *American Journal of Evaluation, 15*(3), 311–319.

Pawson, R., & Tilley, N. (1997). *Realistic evaluation.* SAGE.

Petersen, E. E., Davis, N. L., Goodman, D., Cox, S., Syverson, C., Seed, K., Shapiro-Mendoza, C., Callaghan, W. M., & Barfield, W. (2019). Racial/Ethnic disparities in pregnancy-related deaths—United States, 2007–2016. *Morbidity and Mortality Weekly Report, 68*(35), 762–765. https://www.cdc.gov/mmwr/volumes/68/wr/mm6835a3.htm

Preskill, H., & Boyle, S. (2008). A multidisciplinary model of evaluation capacity building. *American Journal of Evaluation, 29*(4), 443–459.

Preskill, H., & Torres, R. T. (1999). *Evaluative inquiry for learning in organizations.* SAGE.

Proger, A. R., Bhatt, M. P., Cirks, V., & Gurke, D. (2017). *Establishing and sustaining net-worked improvement communities: Lessons from Michigan and Minnesota.* U.S. Department of Education, Institute of Education Sciences, National Center for Education Evaluation and Regional Assistance, Regional Educational Laboratory Midwest. http://ies.ed.gov/ncee/edlabs

Rich, M. (2012, July 23). Enrollment off in big districts, forcing layoffs. *The New York Times.* https://www.nytimes.com/2012/07/24/education/largest-school-districts-see-steady-drop-in-enrollment.html

Rohanna, K. (2017). Breaking the "adopt, attack, abandon" cycle: A case for improvement science in K–12 education. In C. A. Christie, M. Inkelas, & S. Lemire (Eds.), *Improvement science in evaluation: Methods and uses* (New directions for evaluation, vol. 153, pp. 65–77).

Rohanna, K. L. (in press). Extending evaluation capacity building theory to improvement science networks. *American Journal of Evaluation.*

Rohanna, K., & Christie, C. A. (in preparation). *Problem-bound evaluation.*

Rother, M. (2010). *Toyota kata: Managing people for improvement, adaptiveness, and superior results.* McGraw Hill Education.

Russakoff, D. (2014, May 19). Schooled. *The New Yorker.* http://www.newyorker.com/magazine/2014/05/19/schooled

Russ-Eft, D., & Preskill, H. (2009). *Evaluation in organizations* (2nd ed.). Basic Books.

Russell, J., Bryk, A., Dolle, J., Gomez, L., Lemahieu, P., & Grunow, A. (2017). A framework for the initiation of networked improvement communities. *Teachers College Record, 119*(5), 1–36.

Saldaña, J. (2013). *The coding manual for qualitative researchers.* SAGE.

Schön, D. (1983). *The reflective practitioner: How professionals think in action.* Basic Books.

Scriven, M. (1996). Types of evaluation and types of evaluators. *Evaluation Practice, 17*(2), 151–161.

Scriven, M. (1966). The methodology of evaluation. *Social Science Education Consortium, 110.* Purdue University.

Senge, P. M. (2006). *The fifth discipline: The art & practice of the learning organization.* Doubleday.

Senge, P. M., Kleiner, A., Roberts, C., Ross, R. B., & Smith, B. J. (1994). *The fifth discipline fieldbook: Strategies and tools for building a learning organization.* Doubleday.

Senge, P., Kleiner, A., Roberts, C., Ross, R., Roth, G., & Smith, B. (1999). *The dance of change: The challenges of sustaining momentum in learning organizations.* Doubleday.

Sherer, D., Norman, J., Bryk, A. S., Peurach, D. J., Vasudeva, A., & McMahon, K. (2020). *Evidence for improvement: An integrated analytic approach for supporting networks in education.* Carnegie Foundation for the Advancement of Teaching.

Silva, E., & White, T. (May 2013). *Pathways to improvement: Using psychological strategies to help college students master developmental math.* Carnegie Foundation for the Advancement of Teaching. https://www.carnegiefoundation.org/resources/publications/pathways-improvement-using-psychological-strategies-help-college-students-master-developmental-math/

Simpson, D. (2015, May 26). Erno Rubik: How we made Rubik's cube. *The Guardian.* https://www.theguardian.com/culture/2015/may/26/erno-rubik-how-we-made-rubiks-cube

Six Sigma Global Institute. (2020). *Lean Six Sigma: The definitive guide.* https://www.6sigmacertificationonline.com/lean-six-sigma/#Chapter-1-Introduction-and-Background

Six Sigma Global Institute. (2019, October, 25). *What is DMAIC.* https://www.6sigmacertificationonline.com/what-is-dmaic/

Snowden, D. J., & Boone, M. E. (November 2007). A leader's framework for decision making. *Harvard Business Review.* https://hbr.org/2007/11/a-leaders-framework-for-decision-making

Stacey, R. (1996). *Strategic management and organisational dynamics* (2nd ed.). Pitman.

Stroh, D. P. (2015). *Systems thinking for social change: A practical guide to solving complex problems, avoiding unintended consequences, and achieving lasting results.* Chelsea Green.

Teacher Development Trust. (2015). *What is lesson study.* https://tdtrust.org/what-is-lesson-study

Wallop, H. (2014, May 18). Rubik's cube invention: 40 years old and never meant to be a toy. *The Telegraph.* https://www.telegraph.co.uk/technology/google/10840482/Rubiks-cube-invention-40-years-old-and-never-meant-to-be-a-toy.html

Walton, M. (1986). *The Deming management method.* Berkley.

Williams, B. (2015). Prosaic or profound? The adoption of systems ideas by impact evaluation. *IDS Bulletin, 46*(1), 7–16. https://doi.org/10.1111/1759-5436.12117

Williams, B., & Imam, I. (2007). *Systems concepts in evaluation: An expert anthology.* EdgePress.

Williams, C. E. (2015). *Utilizing improvement science to improve population health* [PowerPoint slides]. http://www.ihatoday.org/uploadDocs/1/williamsfull.pdf

Yin, R. K. (2014). *Case study research: Design and methods* (5th ed.). SAGE.

Yurkofsky, M. M., Peterson, A. J., Mehta, J. D., Horwitz-Willis, R., & Frumin, K. M. (2020). Research on continuous improvement: Exploring the complexities of managing educational change. *Review of Research in Education, 44*(1), 403–433. https://doi.org/10.3102/0091732X20907363

Zimmerman, B., & Dooley, K. (2001). *Mergers versus emergers: Rethinking structural change in health care systems.* Working paper, McGill University.

Zimmerman, B., Lindberg, C., & Plsek, P. (1998). *Edgeware: Insights from complexity science for health care leaders.* VHA.

• Index •

Made in United States
Troutdale, OR
03/20/2024

18618230R00100